Handbook of Insomnia

Handbook of Insomnia

Daniel J Taylor
University of North Texas

Philip Gehrman
University of Pennsylvania

Natalie D Dautovich
University of Alabama

Kenneth L Lichstein
University of Alabama

Christina S McCrae
University of Florida

Springer Healthcare

Published by Springer Healthcare Ltd, 236 Gray's Inn Road, London, WC1X 8HB, UK.

www.springerhealthcare.com

British Library Cataloguing-in-Publication Data.

A catalogue record for this book is available from the British Library.

ISBN 978-1-907673-72-6

Project editor: Katrina Dorn
Designer: Roland Codd
Printed in Great Britain by Latimer Trend

Contents

Author biographies

Natalie Dautovich, Ph.D, is an Assistant Professor of Clinical Geropsychology at the University of Alabama. She received her doctorate in Counseling Psychology from the University of Florida and completed a post-doctoral research fellowship at the University of South Florida. Within the area of geropsychology, Dr Dautovich's research focuses on chronopsychology, the study of how our daily activity rhythms, routines, habits, and biological rhythms influence our mental and physical health. Specifically, she has published articles and presented at national conferences on the role of behavioral (daily routines) and biological (sleep) rhythms in the lives of older adults. Also, her research examines the role of these rhythms in response to stress. She relies on intensive, microlongitudinal designs to capture this information.

Philip Gehrman, Ph.D, is an Assistant Professor of Psychology in the Department of Psychiatry of the University of Pennsylvania School of Medicine and a clinical psychologist at the Philadelphia VA Medical Center. He completed his graduate training in clinical psychology at the University of California, San Diego, including a predoctoral internship at the Durham VA Medical Center and a post-doctoral fellowship in sleep medicine at Penn. He has an active research program exploring the mechanisms and treatment of insomnia. Dr Gehrman's clinical work is in the area of behavioral sleep medicine and he provides cognitive behavioral interventions for sleep disorders. Other clinical work includes a national telehealth insomnia program in the Veterans Affairs Health Administration.

Kenneth Lichstein, Ph.D, earned his Ph.D. in child clinical psychology in 1976 at the University of Tennessee, but soon thereafter his interests turned to mid-aged and older adults. He is currently Professor of Psychology, The University of Alabama. He is a fellow of the American Psychological Association and is Certified in Behavioral Sleep Medicine. Early in his career he explored a number of different areas of behavioral medicine including basic psychophysiology, relaxation therapy, anxiety disorders, and headaches. For the past 25 years, his research has focused on sleep with an emphasis on psychological processes in late-life insomnia, hypnotic-dependent insomnia, comorbid insomnia, and epidemiology of sleep. Professor Lichstein's research has been supported continuously since 1988 by the National Institute on Aging, the National Institute on Drug Abuse, the National Institute of Mental Health, private foundations, and industry. He has published over 160 articles/chapters and has authored, coauthored, or co-edited six books. Professor Lichstein has served on the editorial board of a number of journals including the *Journal of Consulting and Clinical Psychology* and *Sleep*. He is the founding editor of the journal *Behavioral Sleep Medicine*, and was a member of the founding Board of Directors of the Society of Behavioral Sleep Medicine.

Christina S McCrae, PhD, CBSM is an Associate Professor in the Dept of Clinical and Health Psychology at the University of Florida, is a licensed clinical psychologist who is certified in behavioral sleep medicine by the American Board of Sleep Medicine. She has received several National Institutes of Health grants to support her research on late life insomnia and insomnia comorbid with medical conditions (fibromyalgia, cardiac disease, gynecologic cancer). Dr McCrae is also the Director of an out-patient insomnia and behavioral sleep medicine clinic at the University of Florida. She is a former president of the Society of Behavioral Sleep Medicine, a member of the executive board of the American Board of Sleep Medicine, an associate editor of *Behavioral Sleep Medicine*, and a former chair of the Insomnia Section of the American Academy of Sleep Medicine.

Daniel J Taylor, PhD, CBSM, D, ABSM is an Associate Professor of Psychology in the Clinical Health Psychology Program at the University of North Texas, where he is also the director of an accredited behavioral sleep medicine training site. Dr Taylor is a licensed psychologist and is certified in both Sleep Medicine and Behavioral Sleep Medicine by the American Board of Sleep Medicine. Dr Taylor has served on the board of directors of the Society of Behavioral Sleep Medicine and Sleep Research

Society and has served on several committees for the American Academy of Sleep Medicine. Dr Taylor has received several National Institutes of Health and Department of Defense grants to support his research on the epidemiology and treatment of insomnia comorbid with medical and psychiatric disorders and has published extensively in these areas.

Chapter 1

Clinical features of insomnia

Definition

Insomnia refers to a difficulty in initiating or maintaining sleep at least three nights per week for at least three months, accompanied by impaired daytime functioning (Table 1.1) [1]. Though not a formal part of the diagnosis, clinicians and researchers also expect to find greater than 30 minutes of sleep onset latency or wake time after sleep onset on poor sleep nights [2]. Chronic, clinically significant insomnia is found in 10% of the population, making it one of the most common psychiatric disorders [3]. It is most often precipitated by stress or a mental disorder, but usually evolves into an independent, self-sustaining problem untethered from the original causal agent [4,5].

Typical insomnia symptoms

Symptom	Characterization
Insomnia identity	Patient believes they have a sleep disorder. Non-complaining poor sleepers (ie, individuals accepting of less than ideal sleep), would not be diagnosed with insomnia.
Difficulty initiating or maintaining sleep	Patient reports it frequently takes more than 30 minutes to fall asleep or awakenings during the night accumulate to more than 30 minutes.
Associated impaired daytime functioning	Patient believes degraded functioning, such as mood disturbance, fatigue, and cognitive impairment, are a by-product of poor sleep. Worry about sleep, during the day and at night, is a common feature of insomnia.

Table 1.1 Typical insomnia symptoms. Adapted from American Psychiatric Association [1] ©American Psychiatric Association.

D. Taylor et al., *Handbook of Insomnia*,
DOI: 10.1007/978-1-907673-73-3_1, © Springer Healthcare 2014

Insomnia conveys a significant burden that can manifest in many ways. Compared to non-affected counterparts, people with insomnia report greater functional disability and greater healthcare utilization [6], experience more injuries [7], and experience an increased incidence of depression and anxiety [8]. More than sleep loss, wakefulness during the night is the most upsetting aspect of the disorder and for many afflicted individuals pervades their nighttime and daytime experience with a dread of bedtime.

Risk factors

Insomnia may occur in any stratum of the population but it is most common in women and older adults [1,3]. Additionally, patients with anxious and worry-prone personality types, increased arousal predisposition, and emotional suppression, may be more susceptible [1]. Environment plays a role, as noise, light, intemperate and uncomfortable surroundings can contribute [1]. Although the strength of the link has not yet been determined, genetics may also act as a risk factor, as insomnia has been shown to have a familial component and higher rates are found in monozygotic twins relative to non-identical twins [1].

Clinical presentation and symptoms of insomnia

Patients with insomnia often do not broach the subject of sleep with their physician unless specifically asked [9]. Those who do present with insomnia will often state that "I just can't sleep." An important aspect of insomnia presentation that needs to be assessed is the portions of the night that are affected by sleeplessness. As such, a difficulty with falling asleep is considered sleep-onset insomnia; waking up in the middle of the night and having difficulty returning back to sleep is considered sleep maintenance insomnia; and waking up early in the morning (ie, earlier than desired) and not being able to return to sleep is considered terminal insomnia or early morning awakenings. These different patterns of insomnia can be helpful for the differential diagnosis of insomnia (discussed in the next section). However, in the majority of cases, patients report that their insomnia affects more than one portion of the night. Over time, an individual's pattern of insomnia can also change [10].

Patients will often present with the daytime complaint of tiredness or fatigue but often do not report being sleepy during the day and it is felt that this is a further manifestation of hyperarousal underlying their insomnia [11]. There are individuals who have difficulty falling asleep or staying asleep at night, but who do not feel that it has any impact on them during the day, and thus will not mention their sleep patterns to their health care providers. Those who seek treatment usually do so because of the perceived negative consequences their insomnia is producing, including cognitive difficulties such as problems with memory, concentration, or decision making. Other presenting daytime complaints include irritability, low energy, and low mood.

Classification

Comprehensive sleep assessment was first introduced in the *Diagnostic and Statistical Manual of Mental Disorders (DSM)* by the American Psychiatric Association [12], and was followed shortly by the first *International Classification of Sleep Disorders (ICSD)* produced by the American Sleep Disorders Association [13]. The most recent revisions of both of these manuals, the fifth edition of the DSM (DSM-5), and the third version of the ICSD (ICSD-3), were coordinated to coincide and reflect better classification uniformity than had been achieved by these two systems in the past [1,14]. Previously, differences between the two systems caused diagnostic confusion in both the clinical and research realms but now the ICSD and DSM-5 criteria closely correspond.

In the DSM-5, clinically significant insomnia is called insomnia disorder and its diagnostic criteria are given in Table 1.2. The criteria require both a complaint of poor sleep and associated daytime impairment, and better accommodate children and dependent older adults than the previous edition. Thus, poor sleep unaccompanied by poor functioning would not qualify as insomnia disorder. The truncated condition might simply be called 'poor sleep' with the patient having symptoms of insomnia. Reserving the formal diagnostic label for those individuals who exhibit the

***Diagnostic and Statistical Manual of Mental Disorders* insomnia criteria**

Criterion	Specification
A. Dissatisfaction with sleep quantity or quality	Complaint by individual (or with children and elderly, complaint by caregiver or family member)
B. Specific symptoms	1. Difficulty initiating sleep; or 2. Difficulty maintaining sleep; or 3. Early-morning awakening 4. In children, bedtime resistance or struggles
C. Distress or impairment	1. Fatigue or low energy 2. Cognitive impairment (eg, attention, concentration, memory) 3. Mood disturbance (eg, irritability, dysphoria) 4. Impaired occupational or academic functioning 5. Impaired interpersonal/social functioning 6. Behavioral problems (eg, hyperactivity, impulsivity, aggression) 7. Negative impact on caregiver or family functioning (eg, fatigue, sleepiness)
D. Frequency	At least 3 nights per week
E. Duration	At least 3 months
F. Opportunity	Adequate opportunity for sleep

Table 1.2 *Diagnostic and Statistical Manual of Mental Disorders* insomnia criteria. Adapted with permission from the American Psychiatric Association [1] ©American Psychiatric Association.

full insomnia syndrome is consistent with consensus insomnia assessment recommendations [15]. The sleep disturbance must occur on average at least three times per week for at least 3 months [14]. The criteria rule out individuals whose poor sleep is attributed to inadequate opportunity due to factors such as demanding work obligations or a disruptive lifestyle.

The ICSD-3 uses the term chronic insomnia disorder (Table 1.3). Like the DSM-5, the ICSD-3 criteria also require both a complaint of poor sleep and associated daytime impairment and accommodate children and dependent older adults. The ICSD-3 adopted the same frequency, duration, and opportunity standards as the DSM-5. The ICSD-3 added a qualifier to account for instances when insomnia is an epiphenomenon of another sleep disorder. For example, if it is determined that the insomnia symptoms do not represent an independent disorder but rather are secondary to obstructive sleep apnea or narcolepsy, this would rule out a chronic insomnia disorder diagnosis.

International Classification of Sleep Disorders insomnia criteria

Criterion	Specification
A. Patient, parent, or caregiver report	1. Difficulty initiating sleep, or 2. Difficulty maintaining sleep, or 3. Early-morning awakening 4. In children, bedtime resistance or struggles
B. Distress or impairment	1. Fatigue/malaise 2. Attention, concentration, or memory impairment 3. Impaired social, family, occupational or academic performance 4. Mood disturbance/irritability 5. Daytime sleepiness 6. Behavioral problems (eg, hyperactivity, impulsivity, aggression) 7. Reduced motivation/energy/initiative 8. Proneness for errors/accidents 9. Concerns about or dissatisfaction with sleep
C. Frequency	At least 3 nights per week
D. Duration	At least 3 months
E. Opportunity	Adequate opportunity for sleep
F. Other sleep disorder	Insomnia complaint is not better explained by another primary sleep disorder

Table 1.3 International Classification of Sleep Disorders insomnia criteria. Adapted with permission from the American Academy of Sleep Medicine [14] ©American Academy of Sleep.

Both the DSM-5 and ICSD-3 have several overlapping symptoms of impaired functioning. Examples of symptoms common to both lists are: fatigue, poor memory, mood disturbance, impaired social or occupational functioning, and hyperactivity, but there are also a few meaningful differences between the two. Unlike the ICSD-3, the DSM-5 identifies the negative impact on caregiver or family functioning as a symptom of insomnia. This would most often apply when a child or dependent older adult has insomnia, but might also be relevant in the case of severe insomnia in any adult. This criterion reflects the impact of insomnia on other members of the household and is a gauge of severity.

Conversely, the ICSD-3 lists three symptoms of impaired functioning that do not appear in the DSM-5: daytime sleepiness, proneness for errors and accidents, and worries about or dissatisfaction with sleep. The daytime sleepiness symptom presumably refers to a subjective complaint, as numerous studies have consistently shown that objective daytime sleepiness does not characterize insomnia [16,17]. Indeed, if objective daytime sleepiness (such as unplanned sleep while watching television or reading) does accompany insomnia, it can imply the comorbid presence of another sleep disorder, such as obstructive sleep apnea. Proneness for errors and accidents is also included in the ICSD-3, which is a well-documented symptom. For example, insomnia unaccompanied by hypnotic use in nursing home residents predicts a 50% increase in falls [18] and insomnia presence confers a two-fold increased risk of injuries in the general population [7]. The third symptom – worry (unwanted intrusive thoughts) about sleep – is a cardinal symptom of insomnia [19]. Worry about sleep not only occurs at bedtime and delays sleep by promoting alertness, but for many individuals it also occurs during daytime, causing anticipatory anxiety. Typical worries about sleep include anticipated sleep difficulty and imagined sleep consequences [20].

The DSM-5 permits supplementing the diagnosis of chronic insomnia with specifiers that add information on associated features of severity, course, duration, and comorbidities. The ICSD-3 include a separate diagnosis, sub-chronic insomnia disorder, which is applied to individuals with a clinically significant disorder that is less frequent or has been in place for a shorter duration than chronic insomnia.

Changes in diagnostic criteria

Insomnia characteristics in the previous version of the DSM (DSM-IV-TR) that have been eliminated in the 2013 version include:

- diagnosis of insomnia related to another mental disorder;
- sleep disorder due to a general medical condition; and
- substance-induced sleep disorder (ie, 'secondary insomnias').

The DSM-5 has added frequency, extended duration, and opportunity criteria [1]. Additionally, the previous version of the ICSD (ICSD-2) specified 11 distinct insomnia diagnoses including: adjustment insomnia, paradoxical insomnia, and inadequate sleep hygiene. However, poor reliability in differential diagnosis justified replacing all of these by the single category: chronic insomnia disorder. The ICSD-3 eliminated the nonrestorative sleep criterion and added frequency and extended duration.

Prognosis

The experience of acute insomnia is typical during periods of life stress or other disruptions to health or routine. For most people, sleep improves once normal patterns are re-established, such as when the source of stress passes or health improves. For others, the insomnia persists and becomes chronic, even in situations in which the initial precipitating factors have passed. These individuals represent the 10% of the US population that suffer from chronic insomnia [3]. There are 25 longitudinal studies conducted at the epidemiologic level that indicate that chronic insomnia, on average, tends to resolve in approximately 45% of cases [10,21–42]. There are several caveats that need to be taken into consideration. First, these studies only assessed insomnia symptoms rather than determining whether clinically significant insomnia was present. This likely led to the inclusion of a number of people with only mild symptoms. In a study by Rosenthal et al that followed patients in a sleep clinic, much lower rates of remission were found [31]. Second, as these studies did not assess insomnia treatment, it is not known whether some of these cases of improvement were due to individuals receiving treatment. Thus, there is a need for more research in this area, but, for now, it is generally thought that while insomnia may improve over time without intervention for some individuals, the majority would benefit from targeted treatment rather than a 'wait-and-see' approach.

References

1 American Psychiatric Association. *Diagnostic and Statistical Manual of Mental Disorders*. 5th edn. Washington, DC: American Psychiatric Association; 2013.

2 Lichstein KL, Durrence HH, Taylor DJ, Bush AJ, Riedel BW. Quantitative criteria for insomnia. *Behavior Res Ther.* 2003;41:427-445.

3 Ohayon MM. Epidemiology of insomnia: what we know and what we still need to learn. *Sleep Med Rev.* 2002;6:97-111.

4 Singareddy R, Vgontzas AN, Fernandez-Mendoza J, et al. Risk factors for incident chronic insomnia: a general population prospective study. *Sleep Med.* 2012;13:346-353.

5 Lichstein K, McCrae C, Wilson N. Secondary insomnia: diagnostic issues, cognitive-behavioral treatment, and future directions. In: Perlis M, Lichstein K, eds. *Treating Sleep Disorders: Principles and Practice of Behavioral Sleep Medicine*. Hoboken, NJ: John Wiley & Sons, Inc.; 2003:286-304.

6 Simon GE, VonKorff M. Prevalence, burden, and treatment of insomnia in primary care. *Am J Psychiatry.*1997;154:1417-1423.

7 Kessler RC, Berglund PA, Coulouvrat C, et al. Insomnia, comorbidity, and risk of injury among insured Americans: results from the America Insomnia Survey. *Sleep.* 2012;35:825.

8 Bolge SC, Joish VN, Balkrishnan R, Kannan H, Drake CL. Burden of chronic sleep maintenance insomnia characterized by nighttime awakenings among anxiety and depression sufferers: results of a national survey. *Prim Care Companion J Clin Psychiatry.* 2010;12.

9 Shochat T, Umphress J, Israel AG, Ancoli-Israel S. Insomnia in primary care patients. *Sleep.* 1999;22 (suppl 2):S359-365.

10 Buysse DJ, Angst J, Gamma A, Ajdacic V, Eich D, Rossler W. Prevalence, course, and comorbidity of insomnia and depression in young adults. *Sleep.* 2008;31:473-480.

11 Benca RM. Consequences of insomnia and its therapies. *J Clin Psychiatry.* 2001;62 (suppl 10):33-38.

12 American Psychiatric Association. *Diagnostic and statistical manual of mental disorders: DSM-III-R.* 3rd edn. Washington, DC: American Psychiatric Association; 1987.

13 American Sleep Disorders Association. *The International Classification of Sleep Disorders: Diagnostic and Coding Manual.* 2nd edn. Westchester, IL: American Academy of Sleep Medicine; 1990.

14 American Academy of Sleep Medicine. *International Classification of Sleep Disorders: Diagnostic and Coding Manual.* 3rd edn. Westchester, IL: American Academy of Sleep Medicine; 2013.

15 Buysse DJ, Ancoli-Israel S, Edinger JD, Lichstein KL, Morin CM. Recommendations for a standard research assessment of insomnia. *Sleep.* 2006;29:1155-1173.

16 Lichstein KL, Wilson NM, Noe SL, Aguillard RN, Bellur SN. Daytime sleepiness in insomnia: Behavioral, biological and subjective indices. *Sleep.* 1994;17:693-702.

17 Stepanski E, Zorick F, Roehrs T, Young D. Daytime alertness in patients with chronic insomnia compared with asymptomatic control subjects. *Sleep.* 1988:54-60.

18 Avidan AY, Fries BE, James ML, Szafara KL, Wright GT, Chervin RD. Insomnia and hypnotic use, recorded in the minimum data set, as predictors of falls and hip fractures in Michigan nursing homes. *J Am Geriatr Soc.* 2005;53:955-962.

19 Harvey AG, Tang NK, Browning L. Cognitive approaches to insomnia. *Clin Psychol Rev.* 2005;25:593-611.

20 Wicklow A, Espie CA. Intrusive thoughts and their relationship to actigraphic measurement of sleep: Towards a cognitive model of insomnia. *Behav Res Therapy.* 2000;38:679-693.

21 Breslau N, Roth T, Rosenthal L, Andreski P. Sleep disturbance and psychiatric disorders: A longitudinal epidemiological study of young adults. *Biol Psychiatry.* 1996;39:411-418.

22 Foley DJ, Monjan AA, Brown SL, Simonsick EM, Wallace RB, Blazer DG. Sleep complaints among elderly persons: an epidemiologic study of three communities. *Sleep.* 1995;18:425-432.

23 Ford DE, Kamerow DB. Epidemiologic study of sleep disturbances and psychiatric disorders. An opportunity for prevention? *JAMA.* 1989;262:1479-1484.

24 Hohagen F, Kappler C, Schramm E, Riemann D, Weyerer S, Berger M. Sleep onset insomnia, sleep maintaining insomnia and insomnia with early morning awakening--temporal stability of subtypes in a longitudinal study on general practice attenders. *Sleep.* Sep 1994;17:551-554.

25 Hohagen F, Rink K, Kappler C, et al. Prevalence and treatment of insomnia in general practice. A longitudinal study. *Eur Arch Psychiatry Clin Neurosci.* 1993;242:329-336.

26 Jansson M, Linton SJ. Psychological mechanisms in the maintenance of insomnia: arousal, distress, and sleep-related beliefs. *Behav Res Ther.* 2007;45:511-521.

27 Katz DA, McHorney CA. Clinical correlates of insomnia in patients with chronic illness. *Archives of Internal Medicine.* 1998;158:1099-1107.

28 Klink ME, Quan SF, Kaltenborn WT, Lebowitz MD. Risk factors associated with complaints of insomnia in a general adult population. Influence of previous complaints of insomnia. *Arch Intern Med.* 1992;152:1634-1637.

29 Livingston G, Blizard B, Mann A. Does sleep disturbance predict depression in elderly people? A study in inner London. *Br J Gen Pract.* 1993;43:445-448.

30 Roberts RE, Shema SJ, Kaplan GA. Prospective data on sleep complaints and associated risk factors in an older cohort. *Psychosom Med.* 1999;61:188-196.

31 Rosenthal LD, Dolan DC, Taylor DJ, Grieser E. Long-term follow-up of patients with insomnia. *Proc (Bayl Univ Med Cent).* 2008;21:264-265.

32 Vollrath M, Wicki W, Angst J. The Zurich study. VIII. Insomnia: association with depression, anxiety, somatic syndromes, and course of insomnia. *Eur Arch Psychiatry Neurol Sci.* 1989;239:113-124.

33 Buysse D, Finn L, Young T. Onset, remission, persistence, and consistency of insomnia symptoms over 10 years: longitudinal results from the Wisconsin Sleep Cohort Study (WSCS). *Sleep.* 2004;27:A268.

34 Ganguli M, Reynolds CF, Gilby JE. Prevalence and persistence of sleep complaints in a rural older community sample: the MoVIES project. *J Am Geriatr Soc.* 1996;44:778-784.

35 Hyyppä MT, Kronholm E, Alanen E. Quality of sleep during economic recession in Finlanc: a longitudinal cohort study. *Soc Sci Med.* 1997;45:731-738.

36 Janson C, Lindberg E, Gislason T, Elmasry A, Boman G. Insomnia in men: a 10-year prospective population based study. *Sleep.* 2001;24:425-430.

37 Jansson-Fröjmark M, Linton SJ. The course of insomnia over one year: a longitudinal study in the general population in Sweden. *Sleep.* 2008;31:881.

38 Jansson-Fröjmark M, Lundquist D, Lundquist N, Linton SJ. *Br J Health Psychol.* 2008;13:121-133.

39 Mendelson WB. Long-term follow-up of chronic insomnia. *Sleep.* 1995;18:698-701.

40 Morin CM, Bélanger L, LeBlanc M, et al. The natural history of insomnia: a population-based 3-year longitudinal study. *Arch Intern Med.* 2009;169:447.

41 Morphy H, Dunn KM, Lewis M, Boardman HF, Croft PR. Epidemiology of insomnia: a longitudinal study in a UK population. *Sleep.* 2007;30:274.

42 Rodin J, McAvay G, Timko C. A longitudinal study of depressed mood and sleep disturbances in elderly adults. *J Gerontol.* 1988;43:P45-P53.

Chapter 2

Causes of insomnia

In this chapter, we will discuss some of the more common factors associated with the development and maintenance of insomnia such as age, physiology, circadian rhythms, and environment.

Age

Aging is one of the most significant factors associated with changes in sleep across the lifetime [1]. Sleep consists of two physiologically distinct states: rapid eye movement (REM) and non-rapid eye movements (NREM) sleep [1]. NREM sleep is associated with minimal mental activity and is divided into three stages, with increasing depth of sleep achieved from stages N1 through N3 (Figure 2.1). REM sleep consists of electroencephalography (EEG) activation, muscle atonia, and rapid eye movements. For most adult sleepers, sleep onset occurs through NREM sleep with REM sleep occurring at least 80 minutes afterwards and NREM and REM sleep typically alternating throughout the rest of the sleeping

Progression of sleep stages across a single night in a normal young adult

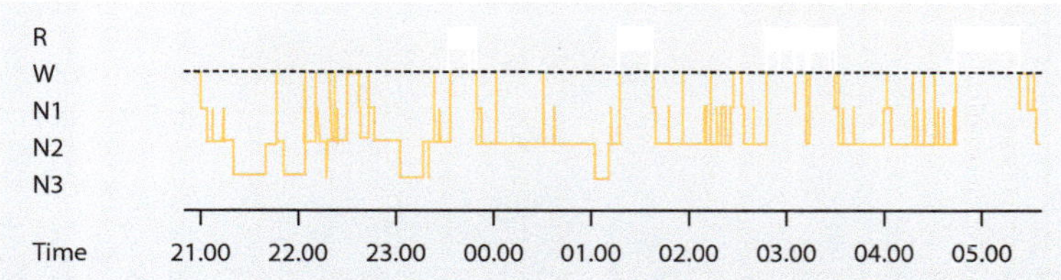

Figure 2.1 Progression of sleep stages across a single night in a normal young adult. (R) Rapid eye movement sleep; (W) Wake; (N1, N2, N3) Non-rapid eye movement sleep stages 1, 2, and 3. Reproduced with permission from Sheenan and Hirshkowitz [2] ©Elsevier.

D. Taylor et al., *Handbook of Insomnia*,
DOI: 10.1007/978-1-907673-73-3_2, © Springer Healthcare 2014

period. REM cycles become longer over time, with a reduction of stage 3 and 4 sleep across the sleep period.

One of the biggest changes in the structure of sleep (also known as 'sleep architecture') is seen in newborn infants. During the first year of life, infants transition from wake to sleep through REM sleep, as opposed to the NREM to REM progression seen in older ages [1]. Infants also begin to develop consolidated nocturnal sleep during their first year of life, with slow wave sleep (also known as 'deep sleep') occurring with the greatest frequency in young children and then decreasing with age [1]. Other age-related changes in sleep (sometimes beginning as early as young adulthood) include an increasing amount of time spent in the lighter stages (ie, N1 and N2) of sleep, more time spent awake, and an advancing of the circadian rhythm (ie, becoming sleepier earlier in the cycle) [1]. Figure 2.2 depicts changes occurring in sleep architecture across the lifespan [3].

Although there are age-related changes in sleep architecture, the majority of changes in sleep are not due to age but rather are a result of various medical and psychiatric comorbidities that become increasingly

Changes in sleep with age

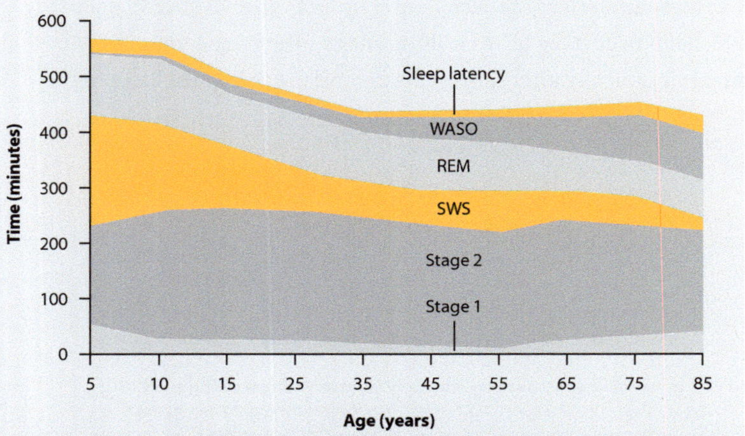

Figure 2.2 Changes in sleep with age. Time (in minutes) for sleep latency and wake time after sleep onset (WASO) and for rapid eye movement (REM) sleep and non-REM (NREM) sleep stages N1, N2, and slow wave sleep (SWS). Summary values are given for ages 5 to 85 years. Reproduced with permission from Ohayon et al [3] ©Associated Professional Sleep Societies.

prevalent with age [1]. As Figure 2.3 illustrates, in addition to factors predisposing older adults to poor sleep, there are a number of factors that can precipitate poor sleep such as the onset of an illness, loss of physical functioning, or another primary sleep disorder (eg, obstructive sleep apnea) [4,5]. Furthermore, once an older adult develops insomnia, there are a number of factors that can perpetuate poor sleep such as social isolation, caregiving, or bereavement.

Understanding the changes in sleep that occur with age is important because older adults may have lowered expectations for their sleep and assume that poor sleep is a natural consequence of aging. As a result, it may be up to the clinician to inquire about sleep complaints from older patients. Poor sleep is an important complaint to assess in older adults as it is associated with poorer overall physical and mental health status [6].

Illustration of the development of sleep complaints and associated adverse outcomes

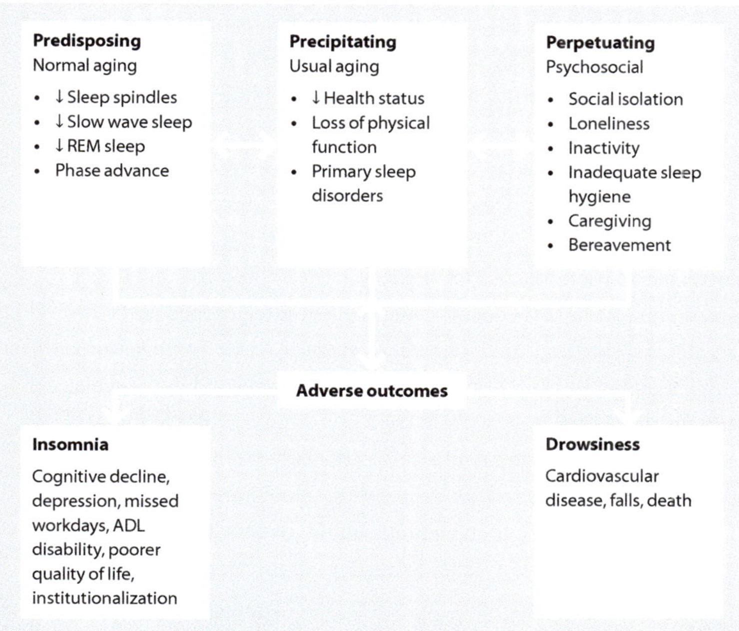

Figure 2.3 Illustration of the development of sleep complaints and associated adverse outcomes. ADL, activities of daily living; REM, rapid eye movement. Reproduced with permission from Vaz Fragoso et al [5] ©John Wiley and Sons.

Specifically, poor sleep has been implicated in an increased risk for falls, impaired physical functioning, cognitive decline, and memory problems in older adults [7–11].

Another consideration for a clinician treating insomnia in older adults is the use of medication. Many medications (eg, anti-hypertensives, inhaled steroids) used in conditions commonly seen in advanced age such as hypertension and chronic obstructive pulmonary disease are known to cause sleep difficulties in older adults. Furthermore, many sedating medications (eg, long-acting benzodiazepines and muscle relaxants) can cause daytime napping that, in turn, could impair nocturnal sleep. Older adults can work with their physician to adjust the dosage or timing of their mediation use to avoid impaired sleep. The effect of medication on sleep architecture will be discussed in more detail later in this chapter.

Additionally, older adults may sometimes employ alcohol as a sleep aid due to its sedating effects. Although initial consumption of alcohol can have a relaxing effect, it can result in a 'rebound' of insomnia, causing the older adult to wake during the night. Accordingly, greater alcohol consumption has been linked to poor sleep in older adults [12,13].

Environmental factors

Several environmental factors can contribute to the development and maintenance of insomnia, including noise, light, temperature, and presence of electronic and communication devices in the bedroom. Individuals with insomnia are often more susceptible to sleep interference and disruption related to external environmental stimuli, such as noise and temperature, than patients without insomnia [14]. Noise and light levels that may not bother other people can have a profound disruptive impact on the sleep of patients with insomnia. For example, external noise from traffic or insects, as well as indoor noises (eg, television, radio, a bed partner's snoring, other people in the household, even a squeaky door hinge) can contribute to a restless and sleepless night for patients with insomnia. Interestingly, white noise or other repetitive noise (eg, sound of a fan) can have a soothing effect and can be conducive to promoting sleep for some patients with insomnia [15,16].

It has been demonstrated that aspects of the bedroom environment, such as the use (or even just the presence) of an electronic device (eg, television, phone) or a desk where finances and/or other paperwork are done, can lead to the bedroom becoming associated with arousing, non-sleep conducive behaviors [17,18]. This may be due to classical conditioning, a theory which helps to explain the importance of 'cues' (ie, discriminative stimuli) in either promoting or disrupting sleep. For patients with normal sleeping patterns, the bed, bedroom, and bedtime are usually strong cues for sleep; inversely, they become strong cues for wakefulness in patients with insomnia, as they adopt and perpetuate arousal-inducing behaviors (eg, worrying, watching TV, surfing the internet, paying bills) while in the bed or bedroom. Another reason for limiting the use of electronic devices in the bedroom is the light from these devices also contributes to arousal.

Another important environmental consideration is how comfortable a patient finds his/her mattress and pillow (eg, size, firmness). For example, patients with insomnia who have comorbid pain and other medical conditions can be greatly impacted by their mattress and pillow, as both impact sleeping position and aggravate pain, which can negatively impact sleep [19–22].

Physiology

Insomnia is generally considered to be a disorder of hyperarousal and the manifestations of this excessive arousal are varied [23]. Initially, investigations focused on somatic hyperarousal in patients with insomnia compared to good sleepers. In these investigations, patients with insomnia were found to have elevations in heart rate, body temperature, galvanic skin conductance, and whole body metabolic rate, all suggestive of elevated activity of the sympathetic nervous system [24,25]. These effects are paralleled by findings that there is elevated activation of the hypothalamic-pituitary-adrenal (HPA) axis in terms of higher levels of cortisol in the blood [26]. These differences seem to be strongest at night and it is as if the body is in a state of 'fight-or-flight,' instead of minimizing arousal in preparation for sleep.

For a number of years, an enigma in the sleep research field was the finding that patients with insomnia often did not have evidence of disturbed sleep during overnight sleep studies when compared to good sleepers, despite feeling that they had slept poorly. One theory about this discrepancy between subjective perceptions and the objective evidence was that there is an inherent limitation in the traditional method of conducting sleep studies [27]. This is because sleep study records are visually scored and so determinations of wake and the different sleep stages rely on direct observation. An alternative approach is to use computer-based spectral analysis measures that decompose the EEG signal into different frequency bands. When this approach was applied to sleep studies of patients with insomnia, it was found that they often display elevated activity in the beta frequency range during sleep [28,29]. Beta EEG activity is usually seen while awake and actively engaged in mental processing. It is now believed that patients with insomnia can experience a state that is a mixture of waking and sleeping features. They appear to be asleep, but at the cortical level they are continuing to process information; this type of 'sleep' is thus perceived as wakefulness. This phenomenon has been referred to as cortical hyperarousal.

Another line of research has been the use of neuroimaging methods to study hyperarousal in insomnia. These studies have been difficult to apply to the study of insomnia, in part due to the loudness of functional magnetic resonance imaging (fMRI) scanners, which often does not allow the patient to undergo scanning while asleep. A few studies have utilized positron emission tomography (PET) imaging in which infusion of the radioisotope can occur during sleep and then the patient can be awoken for scanning [30,31]. These studies have found that, for patients with insomnia and without insomnia, there is a decrease in whole brain arousal in the transition from wakefulness to sleep, as is logical. However, for those with insomnia there is less of a reduction compared to those without (Figure 2.4) [28]. Certain brain regions remain more active during sleep and are another indicator of hyperarousal. One region prone to remaining more active is the reticular activating system, the brainstem region in which most of the major neurotransmitter pathways (eg, serotonin, norepinephrine, acetylcholine, histamine, dopamine, neuropeptide A and B) originate. Given that these neurotransmitters modulate levels of

Functional neuroimaging evidence for hyperarousal in insomnia

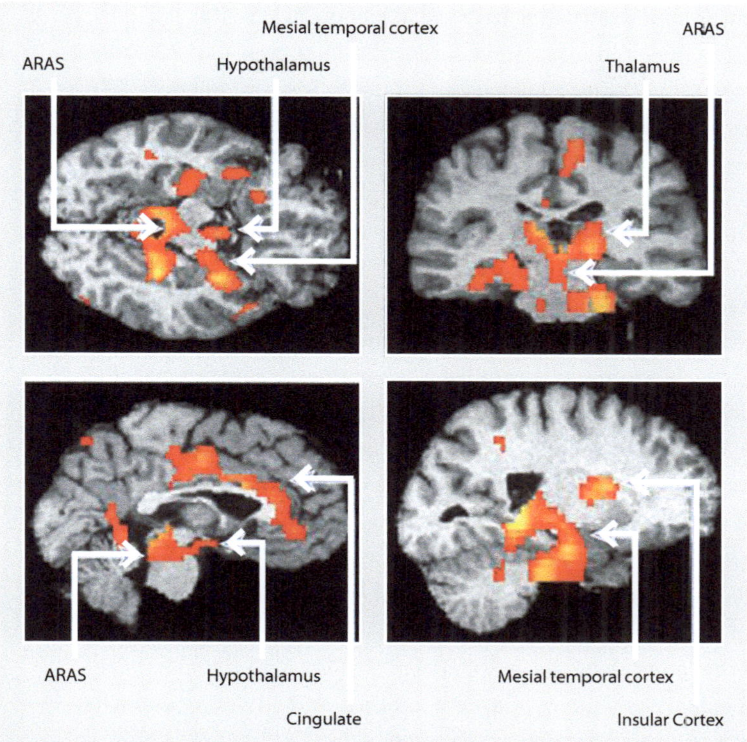

Figure 2.4 Functional neuroimaging evidence for hyperarousal in insomnia. Brain structures that do not show decreased metabolic rate from waking to sleep in patients with insomnia. All regions shown reach statistical significance ($P<0.05$), corrected, level of significance in relation to healthy sleeper control subjects. ARAS, ascending reticular activating system. Reproduced with permission from Nofzinger et al [32] ©American Psychiatric Publishing.

brain arousal, this implies that these systems are maintaining a higher level of arousal in patients with insomnia. It is noteworthy that most sleep medications used to treat insomnia act by way of γ-aminobutyric acid (GABA) mechanisms, as GABA inhibits the activity of the neurotransmitter systems that originate in the reticular activation system. Thus, efficacy of medications used to treat insomnia appears to be due to the ability to reduce brain hyperarousal. Pharmacotherapies are discussed in more detail in Chapter 5.

Circadian rhythms

Circadian rhythms refer to patterning of biological rhythms, including sleep and wake periods, that occur across a 24-hour cycle [33]. Circadian rhythms work with sleep homeostasis to maintain discrete periods of alertness and sleepiness. The two-process model proposed by Borbely describes how the homeostatic (S process) and the circadian process (C process) work in conjunction (Figure 2.5) [34]. Sleep homeostasis refers to the pressure to sleep that accumulates as the duration of wakefulness increases. For example, the homeostatic drive to sleep decreases as the sleep need is met.

Circadian regulation of sleep is not influenced by the amount of preceding sleep, but rather is controlled by an endogenous biological clock located in the suprachiasmatic nucleus (SCN) of the hypothalamus (Figure 2.6) [35,36]. These rhythms typically run longer than 24 hours but they become synchronized to the 24-hour clock via environmental cues (eg, the light–dark cycle). Sunlight is the strongest 'zeitgeber,' or influence, on the timing of sleep and wake. For example, sunlight impacts sleep and wakefulness through its impact on the secretion of melatonin, a hormone which promotes sleep [37]. This is due to sunlight transmitted through the retina along the optic nerve to the SCN in the hypothalamus, which regulates melatonin, body temperature, and other functions that contribute to sleep. Specifically, the pineal gland of the SCN produces melatonin at night (or in darkness), which promotes sleepiness. Thus,

Illustration of the two-process model of sleep regulation

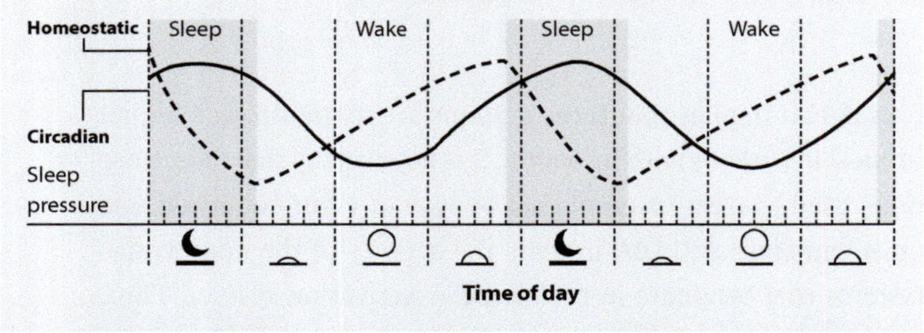

Figure 2.5 Illustration of the two-process model of sleep regulation. Including circadian (solid line) and homeostatic (dashed line) components. Adapted with permission from Borbely [34] and Glickman [35] ©Elsevier.

Pathway light travels through the optic nerve to the areas of the brain that control sleep

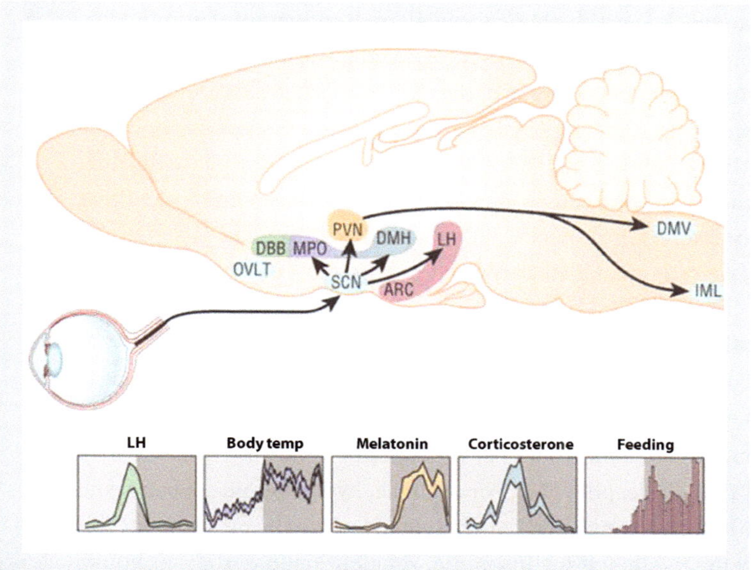

Figure 2.6 Pathway light travels through the optic nerve to the areas of the brain that control sleep. Graphs illustrating the circadian rhythms of luteinizing hormone (LH; involved in ovulation in women and production of testosterone in men), body temperature, melatonin (implicated in the sleep-wake cycle by causing drowsiness and lowering the body temperature), corticosterone (involved in the regulation of immune and stress responses), and feeding in a rat brain. ARC, arcuate nucleus; DBB, double B-box; DMH, wdorsomedial hypothalamic nucleus; DMV, dorsomedial nucleus of vagus; IML, intermediolateral nucleus; MPO, medial preoptic area; OVLT, organum vasculosum lamina terminalis; PVN, paraventricular nucleus; SCN, suprachiasmatic nucleus. Reproduced with permission from Guardiola-Lemaitre and Quera-Salva [37] ©Elsevier.

melatonin production is indirectly inhibited by sunlight and stimulated by darkness. Circadian rhythms complement the homeostatic process by maintaining alertness during day and facilitating sleepiness at night.

Circadian rhythms are implicated in the development of insomnia when there is a mismatch between an individual's internal circadian rhythm and the timing of their sleep-wake cycle. For example, on Sunday night, after staying up late on Friday and Saturday nights, an individual may not experience the onset of sleepiness until midnight. However, because they have to be at work early on Monday, they may attempt to sleep earlier in the evening (eg, 10 PM), and as a result, experience sleep-onset insomnia.

In some cases, the patient may have a circadian rhythm sleep disorder resulting from a significant misalignment between the internal circadian clock and the physical social environment of the individual that is presenting as insomnia [33]. This could be caused by a change in the environment outside of the patient's control, such as shift work or jet lag, or simply that the patient's internal circadian clock does not match that of the 'societal norms,' as seen with advanced sleep phase disorder (ie, circadian rhythm causes significantly earlier sleep and wake times [eg, 8 PM and 2 AM, respectively]) or delayed sleep phase disorder (ie, delayed sleep onset and wake times [eg, 2 AM and 11 AM, respectively]).

Medical conditions and medications

A number of medical conditions (and/or medications that are used to treat them) can impair sleep. As seen in Table 2.1, a variety of medical problems are commonly comorbid with insomnia and may, at least partly, cause difficulty sleeping [38]. For example, hyperthyroidism can result in significant insomnia, and patients should generally be tested for this when being evaluated for insomnia. As mentioned earlier, although insomnia is often precipitated by a medical disorder, the insomnia often decouples and evolves into an independent, self-sustaining problem that can have a reciprocal exacerbation of the medical disorder.

Rates of insomnia in common medical conditions

Disease	Patients with insomnia (%)
Heart disease	44.1
Cancer	41.4
High blood pressure	44.0
Neurological disease	66.7
Breathing problems	59.6
Urinary problems	41.5
Diabetes	47.4
Chronic pain	48.6
Gastrointestinal problems	55.4
Any medical problem	37.8

Table 2.1 Rates of insomnia in common medical conditions. Reproduced with permission from Taylor et al [38] ©Associated Professional Sleep Societies.

Several classes of medications can also cause insomnia. Table 2.2 shows the medications and stimulants that may cause insomnia, with percentage of patients reporting insomnia as a side-effect, when available. The wide variety of insomnia-causing medications indicates that it is always a good idea to review all medications a patient is taking, what the side-effects of those medications are, and when they are taking them (ie, late afternoon administration of stimulating medications is more likely to disrupt sleep than an early morning administration).

Drugs and medications associated with insomnia

Medication	Insomnia incidence (If available)
Central nervous system stimulants	
Amphetamine	
Benzphetamine	
Dextroamphetamine	
Methamphetamine	
Methyphenidate	
Dexmethyphenidate	
Modafinil	
Pemoline	
Phentermine	
Caffeine	
Nicotine	
Psychiatric	
Selective serotonin reuptake inhibitors:	
Fluoxetine	5–9%
Paroxetine	8–14%
Sertraline	7–16%
Citalopram	10%
Escitalopram	9%
Fluvoxamine	15–19%
Other drugs:	
Bupropion	5–19%
Venlafaxine	8%

Table 2.2 Drugs and medications associated with insomnia (continues overleaf). Reproduced with permission from Welsh and Fugit [39] ©John Wiley and Sons.

Drugs and medications associated with insomnia (continued)

Medication	Insomnia incidence (if available)
Respiratory	
Theophylline	1–2%
Aminophylline	
Beta agonists:	
Albuterol	
Metaproterenol	
Terbutaline	
Epinephrine	
Salmeterol	1–2%
Formoterol	
Corticosteroids:	
Prednisone	
Methylprednisolone	
Dexamethasone	
Inhaled corticosteroids	Rare
Antihistamines:	Variable
Bropheniramine	Rare
Diphenhydramine	Rare
Cardiac	
Reserpine	
Diltiazem	
Diuretics:	
Furosemide	
Hydrochlorothiazide	
Bumetanide	
Statins:	
Simvastatin	<1%
Antiarrythmic agents:	
Amiodarone	1–3%
Beta blockers:	Variable
Propranolol	
Metoprolol	
Antimicrobial	
Atovaquone	
Isoniazid	
Meropenem	
Pentamidine	

Table 2.2 Drugs and medications associated with insomnia (continues opposite)

Drugs and medications associated with insomnia (continued)

Medication	Insomnia incidence (if available)
Spectinomycin	
Sulfamethizole	
Sulfasalazine	
Cephalosporins:	
Cefaclor	
Cefpodoxime	
Cefprozil	
Fluroquinolones:	
Ciprofloxacin	1%
Cinoxacin	<1%
Gatifloxacin	2%
Grepafloxacin	>1%
Levofloxacin	0.3%
Ofloxacin	up to 13%
Sparfloxacin	5.7%
Antimalarials:	
Mefloquine	
Antiviral	
Abacavir	12%
Amantadine	14%
Didanosine	22%
Efavirenz	16%
Ganciclovir	5%
Lamivudine	11%
Lopinavir	2%
Ribavirin	
Rimantadine	1–3%
Ritonavir	<2%
Zidovudine	7%
Neurological	
Lamotrigine	6.4%
Felbamate	
Clobazam	
Zonisamide	
Donepezil	6–14%
Baclofen	2–7%

Table 2.2 Drugs and medications associated with insomnia (continues overleaf)

Drugs and medications associated with insomnia (continued)

Medication	Insomnia incidence (if available)
Dopaminergic:	
Levodopa	20%
Entacapone	30%
Amantadine	up to 14%
Endocrine drugs:	
Thyroxine	
Corticosteroids	
Adenocorticotropic hormone (ACTH)	
Gasorelin (in women only)	11%
Tamoxifen	up to 55%
Antineoplastic drugs:	
Vincristine	
Trastuzumab (herceptin, anti-human epidermal growth factor receptor-2)	24–29%
Beta-interferon	>1%
Pamidronate	<1%
Zoledronic acid	>10%
Natural or alternative	
Caffeinated drinks	
• Coffee	
• Black tea	
• Green tea	
Chromium	
Copaiba balsam	
Country mallow	
Cowhage	
Deanol	
Dehydroepiandrosterone (DHEA)	
Ephedra	
Eyebright	
Feverfew	
Ginseng	
• American	
• Panax	
• Panex pseudoginseng	
• Siberian	

Table 2.2 Drugs and medications associated with insomnia (continues opposite)

Drugs and medications associated with insomnia (continued)

Medication	Insomnia incidence (if available)
Guarana	
Khat	
Khella	
Marsh blazing star	
Mate	
Niacin	
Phosphatidylserine	
Policosanol	
SAMe	
St. John's wort	
Sweet vernal grass	
Tiratricol	
Tonka bean	
Valerian	
Vitamin C (ascorbic acid)	
Acerola	
Cherokee rosehip	
Rose hip	
Wormwood (above ground parts)	
Yohimbe	
Withdrawal is associated with rebound insomnia	
Opiates, narcotics	
Barbituates	
Benzodiazepines	
Alcohol	
Gamma-hyroxybutyrate	
Androgenic anabolic steroids	

Table 2.2 Drugs and medications associated with insomnia.

References

1 Carskadon MA, Dement WC. Normal human sleep: an overview. In: Kryger MH, Roth T, Dement WC, eds. *Principles and Practice of Sleep Medicine*. Fifth edn. St. Louis, MO: Elsevier Saunders; 2011:16-26.

2 Keenan S, Hirshkowitz M. Monitoring and Staging Human Sleep. In: Kryger MH RT, Dement WC, ed. *Principles and Practice of Sleep Medicine.* 5th edn. St. Louis, MO: Elsevier Saunders; 2011.

3 Ohayon MM, Carskadon MA, Guilleminault C, Vitiello MV. Meta-analysis of quantitative sleep parameters from childhood to old age in healthy individuals: Developing normative sleep values across the human lifespan. *Sleep.* 2004;27:1255-1273.

4 Spielman AJ, Caruso LS, Glovinsky PB. A behavioral perspective on insomnia treatment. *Psychiatr Clin N Am.* 1987;10:541-553.

5 Vaz Fragoso CA, Gill TM. Sleep complaints in community-living older persons: A multifactorial geriatric syndrome. *J Am Geriatr Soc.* 2007;55:1853-1866.

6 Reid KJ, Martinovich Z, Finkel S, et al. Sleep: a marker of physical and mental health in the elderly. *Am J Geriatr Psych.* 2006;14:860-866.

7 St George RJ, Delbaere K, Williams P, Lord SR. Sleep quality and falls in older people living in self-and assisted-care villages. *Gerontology.* 2008;55:162-168.

8 Blackwell T, Yaffe K, Ancoli-Israel S, et al. Poor sleep is associated with impaired cognitive function in older women: the study of osteoporotic fractures. *J Gerontol A Biol Sci Med Sci.* 2006;61:405-410.

9 Dam TTL, Ewing S, Ancoli-Israel S, Ensrud K, Redline S, Stone K. Association between sleep and physical function in older men: the osteoporotic fractures in men sleep study. *J Am Geriatr Soc.* 2008;56:1665-1673.

10 Goldman SE, Stone KL, Ancoli-Israel S, et al. Poor sleep is associated with poorer physical performance and greater functional limitations in older women. *Sleep.* 2007;30:1317.

11 Foley D, Ancoli-Israel S, Britz P, Walsh J. Sleep disturbances and chronic disease in older adults: results of the 2003 National Sleep Foundation Sleep in America Survey. *J Psychosom Res.* 2004;56:497-502.

12 Dufour MC, Archer L, Gordis E. Alcohol and the elderly. *Clin Geriatr Med.* 1992;8:127.

13 Yao K-W, Yu S, Cheng S-P, Chen I-J. Relationships between personal, depression and social network factors and sleep quality in community-dwelling older adults. *J Nurs Res.* 2008;16:131-139.

14 Jones BT, Macphee LM, Broomfield NM, Jones BC, Espie CA. Sleep-related attentional bias in good, moderate, and poor (primary insomnia) sleepers. *J Abnorm Psychol.* 2005;114:249-258.

15 Richards K, Nagel C, Markie M, Elwell J, Barone C. Use of complementary and alternative therapies to promote sleep in critically ill patients. *Crit Care Nurs Clin North Am.* 2003;15:329-340.

16 Stanchina ML, Abu-Hijleh M, Chaudhry BK, Carlisle CC, Millman RP. The influence of white noise on sleep in subjects exposed to ICU noise. *Sleep Medicine.* 2005;6:423-428.

17 Robertson JA, Broomfield NM, Espie CA. Prospective comparison of subjective arousal during the pre-sleep period in primary sleep-onset insomnia and normal sleepers. *J Sleep Res.* 2007;16:230-238.

18 Brunborg GS, Mentzoni RA, Molde H, et al. The relationship between media use in the bedroom, sleep habits and symptoms of insomnia. *J Sleep Res.* 2011;20:569-575.

19 Colbert AP, Markov MS, Banerji M, Pilla AA. Magnetic mattress pad use in patients with fibromyalgia: a randomized double-blind pilot study. *J Back Musculoskeletal Rehab.* 1999;13:19-31.

20 Kovacs FM, Abraira V, Peña A, et al. Effect of firmness of mattress on chronic non-specific low-back pain: randomised, double-blind, controlled, multicentre trial. *Lancet.* 2003;362:1599-1604.

21 Lavin RA, Pappagallo M, Kuhlemeier KV. Cervical pain: a comparison of three pillows. *Arch Phys Med Rehabil.* 1997;78:193-198.

22 Young G, Jewell D. Interventions for preventing and treating pelvic and back pain in pregnancy. *Cochrane Database Syst Rev.* 2002;(1):CD001139.

23 Riemann D, Spiegelhalder K, Feige B, et al. The hyperarousal model of insomnia: a review of the concept and its evidence. *Sleep Med Rev.* 2010;14:19.

24 Bonnet MH, Arand DL. Heart rate variability in insomniacs and matched normal sleepers. *Psychosom Med.* 1998;60:610-615.

25 Bonnet MH, Arand DL. Situational insomnia: consistency, predictors, and outcomes. *Sleep.* 2003;26:1029-1036.

26 Vgontzas AN, Bixler EO, Lin H-M, et al. Chronic insomnia is associated with nyctohemeral activation of the hypothalamic-pituitary-adrenal axis: clinical implications. *J Clin Endocrinol Metab.* 2001;86:3787-3794.

27 Carskadon MA, Dement WC, Mitler MM, Guilleminault C, Zarcone VP, Spiegel R. Self-reports versus sleep laboratory findings in 122 drug-free subjects with complaints of chronic insomnia. *Am J Psychiatry.* 1976;133:1382-1388.

28 Buysse DJ, Germain A, Hall ML, et al. EEG spectral analysis in primary insomnia: NREM period effects and sex differences. *Sleep.* 2008;31:1673.

29 Perlis ML, Merica H, Smith MT, Giles DE. Beta EEG activity and insomnia. *Sleep Med Rev.* 2001;5:365-376.

30 Nofzinger EA, Nissen C, Germain A, et al. Regional cerebral metabolic correlates of WASO during NREM sleep in insomnia. *J Clin Sleep Med.* 2006;2:316-322.

31 Smith MT, Perlis ML, Chengazi VU, Soeffing J, McCann U. NREM sleep cerebral blood flow before and after behavior therapy for chronic primary insomnia: preliminary single photon emission computed tomography (SPECT) data. *Sleep Medicine.* 2005;6:93-94.

32 Nofzinger EA, Buysse DJ, Germain A, Price JC, Miewald JM, Kupfer DJ. Functional neuroimaging evidence for hyperarousal in insomnia. *Am J Psychiatry.* 2004;161:2126-2128.

33 Reid KJ, Zee PC. Circadian disorders of the sleep-wake cycle. In: Kryger MH, Roth T, Dement WC., eds. *Principles and Practice of Sleep Medicine*. 5th edn. St. Louis, MO: Elsevier/Saunders; 2011:470-482.

34 Borbely AA. A two process model of sleep regulation. *Hum Neurobiol.* 1982;1:195-204.

35 Glickman G. Circadian rhythms and sleep in children with autism. *Neurosci Biobehav Rev.* 2010;34:755-768.

36 Berson DM, Dunn FA, Takao M. Phototransduction by retinal ganglion cells that set the circadian clock. *Science.* 2002;295:1070-1073.

37 Guardiola-Lemaitre B, Quera-Salva MA. Melatonin and the regulation of sleep and circadian rhythms. In: Kryger MH, Roth T, Dement WC, eds. *Principles and Practice of Sleep Medicine.* 5th edn. St. Louis, MO: Elsevier Saunders; 2011.

38 Taylor DJ, Mallory LJ, Lichstein KL, Durrence HH, Riedel BW, Bush AJ. Comorbidity of chronic insomnia with medical problems. *Sleep.* 2007;30:213-218.

39 Welsh CH, Fugit RV. Medications that can cause insomnia. In: Teofilo LC, ed. *Sleep: A Comprehensive Handbook.* New York, NY: Wiley-Liss; 2005:103-109.

Chapter 3

Patient assessment in insomnia

Patient history

There are a number of elements involved in taking a complete patient sleep history. As with any disorder, it is important to determine whether there were any clear precipitants to the insomnia. For example, many patients can identify specific life events or other factors that seemed to trigger their insomnia, although this is not always the case. The temporal course of insomnia over time should be clearly delineated and should include asking about the duration of illness and a determination of whether the course has been constant over time or whether it fluctuates. If the severity changes over time, this may provide clues as to other factors that maintain the insomnia. There should also be an assessment of current frequency of insomnia in terms of the number of nights per week that are affected.

While taking a full medical history is not always necessary for the assessment of insomnia, it is important to consider medical conditions that are likely to affect sleep. In particular, conditions associated with pain, such as osteoarthritis, should be assessed. Patients can often estimate the extent to which their insomnia is solely due to their pain by asking whether the severity of their insomnia correlates with the severity of their pain. Psychiatric disorders are often associated with insomnia, and patients should be asked about any history of mental illness and treatment. Although a detailed psychiatric history may not be necessary, their mood and anxiety levels over the past month should certainly be assessed.

D. Taylor et al., *Handbook of Insomnia*,
DOI: 10.1007/978-1-907673-73-3_3,

If there is a clear history of mental illness, attempts should be made to determine the extent to which the insomnia correlates with episodes of psychiatric disturbance. For example, for a patient with depression, it may be the case that the patient may only have trouble sleeping during depressive episodes.

It can often be helpful to assess the patient's chronotype and their personal circadian rhythms. For example, is the patient more of a 'night owl' (ie, late to sleep, late to wake) by nature or a 'morning person' (ie, early to sleep, early to wake)? Another way to assess chronotype is to ask patients if they tend to follow a different sleep-wake schedule on non-work days or when they are on vacation. If they do indeed follow a very different schedule – and sleep better on that schedule – the underlying problem may be a circadian rhythm disorder rather than insomnia.

Sleep history

A very useful component of assessing a patient's sleep history is to inquire about a typical night of sleep. Considerations to take into account include:

- What is a typical bedtime?
- Do they spend time in bed engaging in other non-sleep activities (eg, reading, watching TV)?
- How long does it typically take to fall asleep (especially once lights are turned off)?
- How many times do they typically wake up during the night?
- Are there particular reasons for waking up (eg, use the bathroom, react to noises)?
- When awoken in the night, how long does it take to get back to sleep?
- What time do they typically wake up for the day?
- Do they wake up on their own or to an alarm clock? If on their own, do they often wake earlier than desired?

The next portion of the sleep history focuses on waking hours and should include a discussion of how they spend their day and the extent to which there is a regular daytime routine. For example, how often and how long does napping occur during the day? It is important to also ask about unintentional dozing (eg, while watching TV) because many patients do not consider this to be 'napping.' Patients should be asked to describe the ways in which their insomnia affects them during the day and what they do to manage this impact.

Sleep hygiene

There should also be a discussion of lifestyle choices and behaviors that may affect sleep (ie, 'sleep hygiene'). For example, this can include documenting caffeine intake, what they consume and at what times of day, as patients are often not aware that teas and sodas contain caffeine, which acts as a stimulant and can disrupt sleep. Use of alcohol, tobacco products, or illicit drugs should also be disclosed, as the closer to bedtime that any of these products are consumed, the more likely they are to affect sleep.

Another aspect of sleep hygiene is the bedroom environment. Patients should be asked to describe their sleep environment in terms of lighting, noise, temperature, and general comfort level (this will be discussed in more detail in Chapter 4). Also, as previously discussed in Chapter 2, excessive light in a room can affect circadian rhythms, including delay if there is too much light in the evening or not enough light in the morning.

It is also important to inquire about a patient's pattern of physical activity. Evidence suggests moderate-to-high intensity exercise 4–8 hours before bedtime results in improved sleep quality in a normal population, but episodes <4 hours and >8 hours before bed results in poorer quality sleep [1–3]. Two studies have shown that a lower level of physical activity or exercise is related to increased risk for insomnia [4,5].

As discussed in Chapter 2, many medications are known to cause insomnia or sedation as side effects. Therefore, patients should be asked to provide a current list of medications that includes both prescribed and over-the-counter (OTC) products, as well as vitamins, herbal, and other dietary supplements. Patients should also be asked about use of recreational substances and OTC products that promote energy, as these products often contain caffeine and their use is growing in popularity. Medications with stimulating or other properties (eg, diuretics) that can also interfere with sleep should be reviewed and potential substitutes with lesser impact on sleep should be considered where appropriate. Likewise, the timing of medications should be considered, as a sleep-interfering medication taken at bedtime may be administered earlier with the same benefit for the target condition but without the negative effect on sleep quality.

Scales and structured interviews

The breadth of areas that need assessment during an insomnia screening (eg, sleep hygiene, medical history, and mental state) are comprehensive enough that it is preferable to perform assessments using some form of structured or semi-structured interview. For example, the Insomnia Interview Schedule (IIS), is a structured interview developed by Morin and published in his landmark book *Insomnia: Psychological Assessment and Management* to provide clinicians with a framework to obtain enough data (eg, symptom severity, sleep-wake schedule, sleep-aid use, history of sleep problems, bedroom environment, diet, exercise, substance use, functional analysis, and comorbid disorder symptoms) to determine a diagnosis in line with major guidelines (eg, *Diagnostic and Statistical Manual of Mental Disorders* [DSM], *International Classification of Sleep Disorders* [ICSD]) [6–8]. However, to date, no structured clinical interview has yet been validated for the assessment of insomnia.

Self-report sleep diaries are essential in the assessment and treatment of insomnia. Numerous versions of sleep diaries are currently available, none of which show superior utility over another. More recently, a consensus sleep diary (Figure 3.1) was developed, but it has yet to be fully verified in clinical trials [9]. Other common self-report measures of insomnia and sleep include the Insomnia Severity Index (ISI) [6], the Pittsburgh Sleep Quality Index (PSQI) [10], the Insomnia Symptom Questionnaire (ISQ) [11], and the Athens Insomnia Scale [12]. Although the PSQI is the most commonly used, it covers a range of other sleep issues (eg, "cannot breathe comfortably," "cough or snore loudly"), and thus is not solely a measure of insomnia and, in some cases, may not be useful as an insomnia-specific measure (eg, ISI) for patients without comorbid conditions. Buysee et al [13] recommends employing standardized measures of contributing domains such as:

- Fatigue: Multidimensional Fatigue Inventory [14] or Fatigue Severity Scale [15];

Consensus sleep diary

Sample								
Today's date	**4/5/11**							
1. What time did you get into bed?	10:15 PM							
2. What time did you try to fall asleep?	11:30 PM							
3. How long did it take for you to fall asleep?	55 minutes							
4. How many times did you wake up, not counting your final awakening?	3 times							
5. In total, how long did these awakenings last?	1 hour, 10 minutes							
6. What time was your final awakening?	6:35 AM							
7. What time did you get out of bed for the day?	7:20 AM							
8. How would you rate the quality of your sleep?	☐ Very poor ☒ Poor ☐ Fair ☐ Good ☐ Very good	☐ Very poor ☐ Poor ☐ Fair ☐ Good ☐ Very good	☐ Very poor ☐ Poor ☐ Fair ☐ Good ☐ Very good	☐ Very poor ☐ Poor ☐ Fair ☐ Good ☐ Very good	☐ Very poor ☐ Poor ☐ Fair ☐ Good ☐ Very good	☐ Very poor ☐ Poor ☐ Fair ☐ Good ☐ Very good	☐ Very poor ☐ Poor ☐ Fair ☐ Good ☐ Very good	☐ Very poor ☐ Poor ☐ Fair ☐ Good ☐ Very good
9. Comments (if applicable)	I have a cold							

Figure 3.1 Consensus sleep diary. Reproduced with permission from Carney et al [9] ©Associated Professional Sleep Societies.

- Depression: Inventory of Depressive Symptomatology [16] or Beck Depression Inventory II [17];
- Anxiety: State-Trait Anxiety Inventory [18]; and
- Quality of life: Short Form Health Survey (SF-36) [19].

Differentiating between secondary contributors and comorbidities

Rates of chronic insomnia are higher in the context of comorbid medical and psychological disorders [20]. In the past, this has led to the rationale that insomnia is a 'symptom' of several medical and psychological disorders (ie, secondary insomnia), and therefore should be resolved through improvement in the primary disorder. However, the factors that precipitate insomnia frequently differ from those that perpetuate and maintain chronic insomnia. Thus, insomnia that begins in response to medical and psychological disorders can become increasingly independent over time, often due to patients acquiring learned and behavioral components that exacerbate and maintain insomnia. At a 2005 National Institutes of Health Consensus Conference on insomnia, experts raised concerns that continuing to view insomnia in the context of medical conditions as 'secondary' in nature (rather than 'comorbid') has resulted in the undertreatment of insomnia [21]. Indeed, several studies have now shown that it is possible to treat insomnia even when comorbid with other medical and psychiatric disorders, with favorable outcomes in both domains [22–27].

Neither polysomnography (PSG; an overnight sleep study), nor actigraphy (a wrist-worn activity monitor that can reliably detect sleep and wake states), is generally recommended for the routine assessment of insomnia [28,29]. However, PSG may be useful when the sleep history reveals symptoms of an underlying sleep disorder (eg, apnea, periodic limb movement disorder [PLMD]), or when insomnia treatments fail [20]. Actigraphy may be useful when the sleep history reveals that symptoms of circadian rhythm disorders are present, or when sleep diaries or single time-point estimates are inappropriate (ie, in residential or low intelligence patient populations) [20].

Sleep apnea is suspected if a patient (or a patient's bed partner) reports heavy snoring, daytime sleepiness, and gasping or choking during the night. Common risk factors of apnea include being >40 years old, male or postmenopausal female, obese, having a large neck (ie, >17 inches for men and >16 inches for women), and craniofacial abnormalities. PLMD is suspected if a patient or their bed partner reports of kicking, jerking during the night, or waking up with very disheveled sheets. It is important to distinguish the typical leg jerks that are normative when falling asleep (often occurring in the transition from wake to sleep) from leg movements that occur throughout the sleep period.

References

1 Youngstedt SD, O'Connor PJ, Dishman RK. The effects of acute exercise on sleep: a quantitative synthesis. *Sleep.* 1997;20:203-214.

2 Singh NA, Clements KM, Fiatarone MA. A randomized controlled trial of the effect of exercise on sleep. *Sleep.* 1997;20:95-101.

3 King AC, Oman RF, Brassington GS, Bliwise DL, Haskell WL. Moderate-intensity exercise and self-rated quality of sleep in older adults. A randomized controlled trial. *JAMA.* 1997;277:32-37.

4 Morgan K. Daytime activity and risk factors for late-life insomnia. *J Sleep Res.* 2003;12:231-238.

5 Sherrill DL, Kotchou K, Quan SF. Association of physical activity and human sleep disorders. *Arch Intern Med.* 1998;158:1894-1898.

6 Morin CM. *Insomnia: Psychological Assessment and Management.* New York, NY: Guilford Press; 1993.

7 American Psychiatric Association. *Diagnostic and Statistical Manual of Mental Disorders.* 5th edn. Washington DC: American Psychiatric Association; 2013.

8 American Academy of Sleep Medicine. *International Classification of Sleep Disorders: Diagnostic and Coding Manual.* 3rd edn. Westchester, IL: American Academy of Sleep Medicine; 2013.

9 Carney CE, Buysse DJ, Ancoli-Israel S, et al. The consensus sleep diary: Standardizing prospective sleep self-monitoring. *Sleep.* 2012;35:287-302.

10 Buysse DJ, Reynolds CF III, Monk TH, Berman SR, Kupfer DJ. The Pittsburgh Sleep Quality Index: A new instrument for psychiatric practice and research. *Psychiatry Res.* 1989;28:193-213.

11 Okun ML, Kravitz HM, Sowers MF, Moul DE, Buysse DJ, Hall M. Psychometric evaluation of the Insomnia Symptom Questionnaire: a self-report measure to identify chronic insomnia. *J Clin Sleep Med.* 2009;5:41.

12 Soldatos CR, Dikeos DG, Paparrigopoulos TJ. The diagnostic validity of the Athens Insomnia Scale. *J Psychosom Res.* 2003;55:263-267.

13 Buysse DJ, Ancoli-Israel S, Edinger JD, Lichstein KL, Morin CM. Recommendations for a standard research assessment of insomnia. *Sleep.* 2006;29:1155-1173.

14 Smets EM, Garssen B, Bonke B, De Haes JC. The Multidimensional Fatigue Inventory (MFI) psychometric qualities of an instrument to assess fatigue. *J Psychosom Res.* 1995;39:315-325.

15 Krupp LB, LaRocca NG, Muir-Nash J, Steinberg AD. The fatigue severity scale. Application to patients with multiple sclerosis and systemic lupus erythematosus. *Arch Neurol.* 1989;46:1121-1123.

16 Rush AJ, Giles DE, Schlesser MA, Fulton CL, Weissenburger J, Burns C. The Inventory for Depressive Symptomatology (IDS): preliminary findings. *Psychiatry Res.* 1986;18:65-87.

17 Beck AT, Steer RA, Ball R, Ranieri WF. Comparison of Beck Depression Inventories-IA and -II in psychiatric outpatients. *J Pers Assess.* 1996;67:588-597.

18 Spielberger CD. *State-trait anxiety inventory: form Y.* Redwood City, CA: Mind Garden; 1983.

19 McHorney CA, Ware JE, Jr., Raczek AE. The MOS 36-Item Short-Form Health Survey (SF-36): II. Psychometric and clinical tests of validity in measuring physical and mental health constructs. *Med Care.* 1993;31:247-263.

20 Schutte-Rodin S, Broch L, Buysse D, Dorsey C, Sateia M. Clinical guideline for the evaluation and management of chronic insomnia in adults. *J Clin Sleep Med.* 2008;4:487-504.

21 National Institutes of Health. National Institutes of Health State of the Science Conference statement on Manifestations and Management of Chronic Insomnia in Adults, June 13-15, 2005. *Sleep.* 2005;28:1049-1057.

22 Manber R, Edinger JD, Gress JL, San Pedro-Salcedo MG, Kuo TF, Kalista T. Cognitive behavioral therapy for insomnia enhances depression outcome in patients with comorbid major depressive disorder and insomnia. *Sleep.* 2008;31:489-495.

23 Savard J, Simard S, Ivers H, Morin CM. Randomized study on the efficacy of cognitive-behavioral therapy for insomnia secondary to breast cancer, part I: Sleep and psychological effects. *J Clin Oncol.* 2005;23:6083-6096.

24 Rybarczyk B, Stepanski E, Fogg L, Lopez M, Barry P, Davis A. A placebo-controlled test of cognitive-behavioral therapy for comorbid insomnia in older adults. *J Consult Clin Psychol.* 2005;73:1164-1174.

25 Edinger JD, Olsen MK, Stechuchak KM, et al. Cognitive behavioral therapy for patients with primary insomnia or insomnia associated predominantly with mixed psychiatric disorders: a randomized clinical trial. *Sleep.* 2009;32:499.

26 Brower KJ, Myra Kim H, Strobbe S, Karam-Hage MA, Consens F, Zucker RA. A randomized double-blind pilot trial of gabapentin versus placebo to treat alcohol dependence and comorbid insomnia. *Alcohol Clin Exp Res.* 2008;32:1429-1438.

27 Pollack M, Kinrys G, Krystal A, et al. Eszopiclone coadministered with escitalopram in patients with insomnia and comorbid generalized anxiety disorder. *Arch Gen Psychiatry.* 2008;65:551.

28 Littner M, Hirshkowitz M, Kramer M, et al. Practice parameters for using polysomnography to evaluate insomnia: an update. *Sleep.* 2003;26:754-760.

29 Littner M, Kushida CA, Anderson WM, et al. Practice parameters for the role of actigraphy in the study of sleep and circadian rhythms: an update for 2002. *Sleep.* 2003;26:337-341.

Chapter 4

Treating insomnia

Lifestyle adjustments

Treatment of insomnia is virtually always initiated by a patient complaint, and adequate resolution is nearly always determined by patient-reported outcomes, revealing the crucial role of patient participation and perception in insomnia. Accordingly, lifestyle adjustments are often crucial for successful treatment and prevention of insomnia. This includes, but is not limited to, proper sleep hygiene, a group of psycho-educational lifestyle adjustments designed to address a variety of behaviors that may affect sleep [1]. The most common instructions are to avoid exercise, large meals, excessive fluids, nicotine and alcohol within 2 hours of bedtime; avoid caffeine within 6 hours of bedtime; and create a sleep environment that is cool, dark, quiet, and comfortable. Clinicians sometimes confuse sleep hygiene and stimulus control because the instructions are similar and often combined. Although generally considered a good adjunctive addition to sleep restriction, stimulus control, relaxation therapy, and cognitive behavioral therapy (CBT), sleep hygiene has not been proven to be efficacious as a stand-alone treatment [2,3]. This is most likely because the instructions are not relevant for people with chronic insomnia who are already practicing good sleep hygiene.

There is increasing interest in what is referred to as 'social rhythmicity' (eg, social activities, timing of meals, and other daytime activities) and its impact on sleep [4–7]. For example, providing a structured schedule of social and physical activities for residents of an assisted living facility

D. Taylor et al., *Handbook of Insomnia*,
DOI: 10.1007/978-1-907673-73-3_4, © Springer Healthcare 2014

resulted in increased amounts of slow-wave sleep and improvement on memory tasks [4]. Although additional research is needed, recommending greater regularization in mealtimes and increased regular social interaction is not likely to negatively interfere with sleep and is likely to have a positive impact on mood (specifically social interaction), which can positively impact sleep.

Another lifestyle adjustment that may also positively impact sleep is regular exercise. It has been suggested that exercising too close to sleep initiation can contribute to arousal that interferes with sleep but exercising earlier in the day may have a positive impact [8]. For instance, exercising with exposure to natural sunlight earlier in the day can help to inhibit melatonin production to promote daytime wakefulness (as increased melatonin contributes to sleepiness [9]).

Behavioral therapy

Behavioral interventions for insomnia (ie, stimulus control therapy, sleep restriction, and progressive muscle relaxation) are all considered empirically validated treatments and are generally based on the behavioral model of insomnia [10]. They are often combined with sleep education, sleep hygiene, and cognitive interventions into multi-modal CBT for insomnia. Research has shown that behavioral interventions alone, or in combination with cognitive therapy and sleep hygiene, can be used to effectively treat both primary insomnia and insomnia comorbid with other disorders [3,11–16]. They are as effective as medications in the short-term and have better long-term outcomes than medication [17–20]. This is discussed in more detail in Chapter 5.

Stimulus control

Stimulus control instructions are based on the theory that insomnia is perpetuated by repeated association of the bedroom with poor sleep, as well as worrying, planning, or recreation. Patients are therefore told to use the bed only for sleep in an attempt to extinguish the maladaptive associations [21]. The most common stimulus control instructions are to:

- Step 1: do not use the bed or bedroom for anything but sleep (or sex);
- Step 2: go to bed only when ready to sleep;

- Step 3: leave the bed and do something in another room if sleep onset is greater than 15 minutes;
- Step 4: return to bed only when feeling a strong sleep urge;
- Step 5: if you do not fall asleep quickly upon returning to bed, start over at Step 3 as many times as is necessary;
- Step 6: use an alarm to awaken at the same time every morning; and
- Step 7: do not nap during the day.

In order to avoid using the bedroom, patients are often told to remove everything from their room not associated with sleep, such as the TV, desk, and computer.

Sleep restriction

Sleep restriction is based on the theory that people who develop acute insomnia cope by spending too much time in bed, which then perpetuates insomnia into a chronic disorder. Patients are, therefore, told to reduce total time in bed to more accurately reflect the amount of time they spent sleeping on a typical night [10]. Thus, if a patient spends 10 hours in bed per night to get an average of 5.5 hours of sleep, their sleep schedule is modified so that the patient will only spend a total of 5.5 hours in bed. As patient's total sleep time improves with treatment (ie, sleep efficiency >87%), their sleep schedule is increased (typically 15 min per week) [10]. There are variations of this treatment (eg, sleep schedule = average sleep time + 30 minutes; increase when sleep efficiency >90%), but most practitioners set 5 hours as the minimum target sleep schedule. An alternative approach is sleep compression, where reduction in time in bed is done incrementally (eg, 15–30 minutes per session) [22]. This approach can sometimes decrease patient anxiety about losing sleep.

Relaxation therapy

Relaxation therapy is based on the theory that people with insomnia have elevated levels of physiological and mental arousal that can inhibit sleep. Patients are, therefore, taught relaxation procedures that they can practice on their own to counteract this. Several relaxation interventions and variations exist (eg, imagery, meditation, biofeedback). For example, progressive muscle relaxation (PMR) involves patients alternating between tensing and relaxing different muscle group throughout the body for approximately 20–45 seconds [23,24]. The PMR process typically takes 10–30 minutes per session, depending on the method used. Patients often need several weeks to master this skill and thus are encouraged to practice two times daily, once during the day and once at bedtime.

Cognitive therapy

How an individual thinks about their sleep can have an impact on how well they sleep. As such, negative cognitions or thought patterns (also referred to as dysfunctional or maladaptive thoughts) can produce arousal that interferes with sleep. A cognitive model of insomnia (Figure 4.1) posits that patients with insomnia tend to 'over focus' on sleep and have distorted beliefs about sleep and its impact on daytime performance [25].

These thought processes contribute to a spiraling increase of negative thoughts that result in more worry and arousal (both physiological and emotional) and, subsequently, the development and maintenance of chronic insomnia. For example, patients can develop negative, sleep-related thought patterns related to their frustration over their inability to sleep and overly negative interpretations/perceptions of the negative impacts of poor sleep. Common types of negative thought patterns include distorted beliefs about one's ability to sleep (ie, starting to think that one will never sleep well again), over focus on well popularized ideals (ie, "I need 8 hours of sleep, because that's the amount everyone needs"), and concerns about the impact of sleep on health (ie, "My cancer may come out of remission if I don't start getting more sleep soon"). Sometimes the thoughts that interfere with sleep are not directly related to sleep. Instead, patients may worry about other aspects of their lives, including finances, relationships, and work performance. Table 4.1 lists examples of common sleep-interfering thoughts as assessed by the Dysfunctional Beliefs and Attitudes About Sleep scale [26].

Cognitive therapy directly targets sleep-interfering thoughts, regardless of whether the thoughts are sleep-specific or more general arousal-inducing types of thoughts that occur near bedtime. Cognitive therapy involves several steps. First, the clinician works with the patient to identify

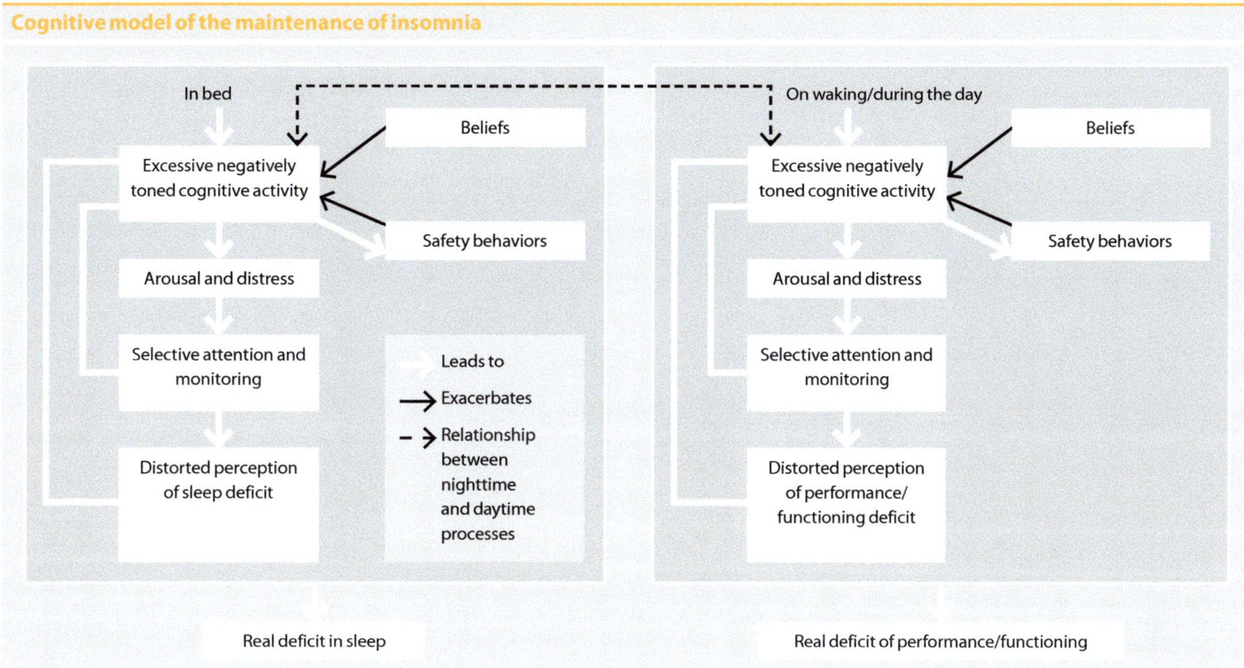

Figure 4.1 Cognitive model of the maintenance of insomnia. This figure describes how pervasive, negatively-toned cognitions about impaired sleep and daytime functioning trigger autonomic arousal and emotional distress, eventually leading the individual to overestimate the extent of their perceived deficits. Reproduced with permission from Harvey [25] © Elsevier.

Dysfunctional Beliefs and Attitudes About Sleep Scale

- I need 8 hours of sleep to feel refreshed and function well during the day.
- When I don't get the proper amount of sleep on a given night, I need to catch up on the next day by napping or on the next night by sleeping longer.
- I am concerned that chronic insomnia may have serious consequences on my physical health.
- I am worried that I may lose control over my abilities to sleep.
- After a poor night's sleep, I know that it will interfere with my daily activities on the next day.
- In order to be alert and function well during the day, I believe I would be better off taking a sleeping pill rather than having a poor night's sleep.
- When I feel irritable, depressed, or anxious during the day, it is mostly because I did not sleep well the night before.
- When I sleep poorly on one night, I know it will disturb my sleep schedule for the whole week.
- Without an adequate night's sleep, I can hardly function the next day.
- I can't ever predict whether I'll have a good or poor night's sleep.
- I have little ability to manage the negative consequences of disturbed sleep.
- When I feel tired, have no energy, or just seem not to function well during the day, it is generally because I did not sleep well the night before.
- I believe insomnia is essentially the result of a chemical imbalance.
- I feel insomnia is ruining my ability to enjoy life and prevents me from doing what I want.
- Medication is probably the only solution to sleeplessness.
- I avoid or cancel obligations (social, family) after a poor night's sleep.

Each of these thoughts are measured on a sliding scale from 0 (strongly disagree) to 10 (strongly agree)

Strongly disagree	**0**	**1**	**2**	**3**	**4**	**5**	**6**	**7**	**8**	**9**	**10**	**Strongly agree**

Table 4.1 Dysfunctional Beliefs and Attitudes About Sleep Scale. Adapted with permission from Morin et al [26] ©Guildford Press.

their sleep-interfering thoughts. Home recording of such thoughts, when/where they occur, and the specific negative emotions (and the level of that emotion on a 0–100 point scale) experienced while thinking them is often conducted to capture a patient's most frequent and distressing thoughts. An example of this, known as a thought record, is seen in Figure 4.2 [27]. This exercise teaches a patient to begin noticing these types of thoughts and their relationship to negative emotions and poor sleep.

The next step involves challenging the validity of those thoughts and replacing them with more sleep-conducive thoughts (ie, more functional

Thought record for cognitive therapy

Situation	Mood (intensity 0–100%)	Thoughts	Evidence *for* the thought	Evidence *against* the thought	Adaptive/ coping statement	Do you feel any differently?

Figure 4.2 Thought record for cognitive therapy. Reproduced with permission from Edinger and Carney [27] ©Oxford University Press.

or adaptive ones). For example, a more sleep-conducive thought for a dysfunctional belief could be:

"I may feel a little more tired following a bad night's sleep, but that's normal for everyone, including cancer survivors. After a poor night's sleep, I can make sure I engage in other health behaviors the following day. Also, I can learn new strategies to help improve my sleep and allow me to cope with fluctuations in my sleep."

As the patient identifies, challenges, and replaces these negative thoughts and beliefs, their arousal levels decrease, and sleep improves. Cognitive therapy is typically used in combination with other empirically validated treatments (ie, stimulus control, sleep restriction, progressive muscle relaxation) because research has yet to establish its efficacy and effectiveness as a stand-alone treatment [2,3].

Pharmacotherapy

Two major consensus papers have been written to help guide decision making with regards to pharmacotherapy for insomnia, as well as a clinical guidelines manuscript [28–30]. They are all in agreement that cognitive therapy is effective and should be offered as a first-line intervention where available [28–30]. However, pharmacotherapy is still the most commonly used treatment for insomnia, although it should be supplemented with behavioral and cognitive therapies where possible [28]. Pharmacotherapy requires health care providers and patients alike to exercise caution due to a risk of dependence and residual daytime impairment. Three main classes of medications are currently used to treat insomnia: benzodiazepine receptor agonists (BzRAs), non-benzodiazepine hypnotics, and antidepressants. Older drugs such as barbiturates are rarely used today and are not recommended because of their many detrimental side effects [28].

Benzodiazepine receptor agonists

Gamma-Aminobutyric acid (GABA) is the primary inhibitory neurotransmitter in the central nervous system of mammals, and GABAergic projections appear to inhibit monoaminergic arousal centers in the brain. There are two primary GABA receptors: $GABA_A$ and $GABA_B$. With regards to insomnia, $GABA_A$ receptors have been the primary target because they appear to control sedation and muscle relaxation. $GABA_A$ receptors have five subunits on the core anion channel that differ in both their distribution and properties, and combine to form combinations of subtypes of receptors. The most abundant subtypes are α1β2γ2, α2β3γ2, and α3β3γ2. The -γ2 subunits (85% of $GABA_A$ subtypes) are widely dispersed and have more sedative, amnestic, anticonvulsant, and anxiolytic effects. The subtypes with α1-subunits (60%) are primarily distributed in the thalamic and cortical areas and are associated primarily with sedating, amnestic, and anticonvulsant effects. The differences between the various GABAergic drugs developed for the treatment of insomnia resides in the different sensitivity the $GABA_A$ receptor subtypes have for the medications.

BzRAs (Table 4.2) are a class of drugs that have equivalent affinity with all $GABA_A$-γ2 receptors. BzRAs were considered the hypnotics of choice for treating insomnia because they resulted in reduced sleep onset latency and wake time after sleep onset, increasing total sleep time and continuity, were less lethal than barbiturates in overdose and were thought to be non-addictive [28]. However, evidence eventually demonstrated that BzRAs are associated with tolerance, rebound insomnia upon withdrawal, and daytime residual effects (eg, amnesia and risk for falls in older adults, cognitive difficulties, and daytime fatigue). Thus, most formulations are no longer recommended for treatment of insomnia, especially in people over 60 years of age [31]. However, short-acting

Pharmacotherapy options: benzodiazepine receptor agonists

Drug	Dosage form	Recommended dosage (mg hs)	Half-life (hours)	Indications/ specific comments
Estazolam	1,2 mg tablets	1–2; 0.5 in elderly or debilitated	8–24	Short- to intermediate-acting
Temazepam	7.5, 15, 30 mg capsules	15–30; 7.5 elderly or debilitated	8–20	Short- to intermediate-acting
Triazolam	0.125, 0.25 mg tablets	0.25 (max 0.5); 0.125 in elderly or debilitated; (max 0.25)	2–6	Short-acting
Flurazepam	15, 30 mg capsules	15–30; 15 in elderly or debilitated	48–120	Long-acting; Risk of residual daytime drowsiness

Table 4.2 Pharmacotherapy options: benzodiazepine receptor agonists. hs, at bedtime. Adapted with permission from Schutte-Rodin et al [28] ©American Academy of Sleep Medicine.

BzRAs (eg, triazolam, temazepam) are acceptable for use, although not generally recommended [28,29].

Non-benzodiazepine hypnotics

Newer non-benzodiazepine (Table 4.3) drugs are more specific in their receptor affinity, primarily on $GABA_A$ α1-subunit receptors, reducing the number of receptors by approximately 25%. These new compounds are said to be non-addictive and have fewer side effects (primarily next day sedation) than BzRAs, due in part to the more selective receptor affinity as well as shorter half-life [32]. These drugs still may result in dependence and are classified by the US Food and Drug Administration (FDA) as Schedule IV controlled substances due to the potential for abuse or dependence, primarily in individuals with a history of abuse or dependence and those with a history of psychiatric diseases [33]. In addition, reports of negative side effects have begun to surface recently, including rebound insomnia, subjective ratings suggestive of abuse potential, anxiety, sleep-related eating disorder, and short-term memory decrements [34]. These increases in risk have prompted the FDA to request that all manufacturers of sedative-hypnotic drugs strengthen their product labeling regarding

Pharmacotherapy options: non-benzodiazepine hypnotics.

Drug	Dosage form	Recommended dosage (mg hs)	Half-life (hours)	Indications/ specific comments
Cyclopyrrolones				
Eszopicione	1, 2, 3 mg tablets	2–3; 1 in elderly or debilitated (max 2); 1 in severe hepatic impairment (max 2)	6	Primarily used for sleep-onset and maintenance insomnia; intermediate-acting; no short-term usage restriction
Imidazopyridines				
Zolpidem	5, 10 mg tablets	10 (max 10); 5 in elderly, debilitated, or hepatic impairment	2–3	Primarily used for sleep-onset insomnia; short- to intermediate-acting
Zolpidem (controlled release)	6.25, 12.5 mg tablets	12.5; 6.25 in elderly, debilitated, or hepatic impairment	3–4	Primarily used for sleep-onset and maintenance insomnia; controlled release; swallow whole, not divided, crushed or chewed
Pyrazolopyrimidines				
Zaleplon	5, 10 mg tablets	10 (max 20); 5 in elderly, debilitated, or hepatic impairment	1–2	Primarily used for sleep-onset insomnia; maintenance insomnia as long as 4 hours is available for further sleep; short-acting

Table 4.3 Pharmacotherapy options: non-benzodiazepine hypnotics. hs, at bedtime. Adapted with permission from Sharon Schutte-Rodin et al [28] © American Academy of Sleep Medicine.

potential for risks to include severe allergic reactions and complex sleep-related behaviors, which may include sleep-driving [33].

Zolpidem

Zolpidem is the oldest nonbenzodiazepine hypnotic and has been proven to be effective in improving sleep-onset latency and total sleep time, but not middle-of-the-night awakenings [35–38]. Recent open-label trials have shown that this medication does not result in rebound insomnia after 12 months' use [39]. Patients who take zolpidem should not be active for at least 7 to 8 hours after taking the medication. A controlled-release (CR) formulation has been developed to help with patients who have middle-of-the-night or early morning awakenings, and has been shown to be effective at 12.5 mg for up to 12 months [40]. Newer, faster acting preparations have been developed that come in oral mist and sublingual forms [41–43]. In January of 2013, the FDA required lower doses of all versions of zolpidem recommended for women (6.25 mg of extended-release, 5 mg of immediate-release) because women take longer than men to eliminate the medication from their blood, resulting in increased risk of side effects such as next-day impairment and drowsiness [44].

Zaleplon

Zaleplon is a compound with a very short half-life (1–2 hours), which makes it appropriate for both sleep-onset difficulties and middle-of-the-night insomnia. It is also used for treating maintenance insomnia or early morning awakenings, as long as the patient does not plan to get out of bed for another 4 hours. In a double-blind, parallel-group, placebo-controlled study, polysomnographic and subjective sleep data were collected over two nights per week for 5 weeks and on the first two nights after discontinuation of active medication. Zaleplon was shown to be effective for significantly reducing sleep latency when compared to placebo, but not total sleep time, for up to 5 weeks of treatment without resulting in rebound insomnia [45]. These results were replicated in a study of older adults over two weeks [46].

Eszopiclone

Eszopiclone is one of the newest members of this class and has been shown to improve sleep-onset latency, wake time after sleep onset, and total sleep time [47,48]. The medication has also shown hypnotic efficacy for as long as 6–12 months [47,48]. In the 6-month open-label extension phase of a 6-month randomized, double-blind, placebo-controlled study, patients initially randomized to placebo and then switched to open-label eszopiclone significantly reported decreased sleep latency, wake time after sleep-onset, and number of awakenings; increased total sleep time and sleep quality; and improved ratings of daytime ability to function, alertness, and sense of physical well-being compared to baseline ($P \leq 0.0001$)[48]. Eszopiclone has also been shown to improve response to antidepressant medications in patients with both insomnia and depression [49].

Melatonin receptor agonists

Ramelteon

Ramelteon is a relatively new hypnotic that does not act on the GABA receptors, but instead, is a melatonin receptor agonist, with high affinity for MT_1 and MT_2 subtypes. Melatonin helps regulate the circadian clock and is normally secreted during periods of darkness, which typically corresponds with sleep in humans. Melatonin can induce sedation, which may result through lowering of body temperature or some other unknown mechanism. In a randomized, multicenter, double-blind, placebo-controlled trial of nightly ramelteon treatment (8 mg or 16 mg) in adults with primary chronic insomnia, ramelteon was found to improve latency to persistent sleep and total sleep time when compared to placebo for up to 6 months [50]. The most common adverse event was headache (19.4% for 8 mg; 17.8% for 16 mg). This is the only drug in this class that is not listed as a controlled substance, as it shows little-to-no potential for abuse, because rebound insomnia and withdrawal effects are not seen after discontinuation following chronic use [50].

Antidepressants

Tricyclic antidepressants (TCAs), in smaller dosages than normally used for depression, are the most common antidepressants used off-label as insomnia medications (Table 4.4), despite only one (doxepine), having approval by the FDA for such use [51]. TCAs act on a variety of receptors throughout the body, but the primary site of activity for insomnia is histamine-1 receptors as antagonists, which reduces arousal. Data from studies on the effect of TCAs on insomnia show these drugs have mixed effects on sleep latency, total sleep time, and number of awakenings [52]. Studies have found that, unlike BzRAs, antidepressant medications have almost no abuse potential because dosages do not need to be continually increased to remain effective and they do not produce withdrawal symptoms when stopped [53]. Trazodone appears to be the most effective, but the effectiveness was not proven to last longer than 1 week [36]. To date, only low-dose (25 mg) doxepine has been approved for use in insomnia, with efficacy for up to 5 weeks for reducing wake time after sleep onset, while increasing total sleep time and sleep efficiency [54].

Nonprescription treatments

Commonly used nonprescription treatments for insomnia are often over-the-counter (OTC) 'sleep aids' (ie, antihistamines such as doxylamin and diphenhydramine), and nonsteroidal anti-inflammatory drugs (eg, acetaminophen) with antihistamines included (eg, "PM" drugs). OTC products have not been as well studied as prescription treatments, and evidence demonstrating efficacy, side effects, and potential for tolerance and dependence is lacking [55,56]. However, data suggest that tolerance

Antidepressants commonly used in insomnia

Drug	Dosage (mg)	Half-life (hr)
Amitriptyline	25–150	5–45
Doxepine	10–100 (generic); 3–6 (proprietary)	10–30
Nefazodone	50–150	6–18
Sinequan	25–150	10–30
Trazodone	25–150	3–14

Table 4.4 Antidepressants commonly used in insomnia.

to antihistamines develops in as little as 4 days and they should not be recommended as a treatment for insomnia [57].

Herbal OTC remedies commonly used by insomnia patients (eg, melatonin and valerian) have very little research backing them and no FDA oversight, so it is difficult to determine quality between manufacturers. In two studies that examined efficacy, neither melatonin nor valerian was significantly better at improving sleep than placebo [58,59].

Emerging treatments

Suvorexant

Orexin is a neurotransmitter that appears to promote wakefulness through excitation of dopamine, norepinephrine, histamine, and acetylcholine systems. Genes for orexin appear to be mutated or missing in animals and humans with narcolepsy, and sleep deprivation increases levels of orexin in the body. Suvorexant is a dual orexin receptor antagonist which appears to improve sleep efficiency by inhibiting wakefulness, rather than by inducing sleep, via orexin receptor-1 and orexin receptor-2 antagonism [60,61]. In two pivotal randomized, double-blind, placebo-controlled, crossover studies, patients with primary insomnia who received suvorexant showed dose-related improvements, including improved sleep latency and sleep maintenance, when compared to placebo [61]. Patients given suvorexant reported a reduction in the time it took for them to fall asleep, as well as staying asleep for longer (60.3 minutes longer vs 40.6 minutes with placebo). Additionally, polysomnographic measures were also used in the study and patients given suvorexant entered into continuous sleep faster and spent less time awake during the night [60]. No pattern of rebound insomnia or withdrawal effects was observed after 4 weeks of treatment. The FDA in the US recently determined that suvorexant is generally safe and effective for treating insomnia, recommending starting doses of 15 mg for elderly and 20 mg for non-elderly but noted concerns regarding evidence of increased daytime sleepiness and suicidal ideation at higher doses.

Tasimelteon

Tasimelteon is a novel MT_1 and MT_2 agonist with high affinity for human melatonin receptors that is currently being investigated for sleep disorders. In a recent Phase III study, 411 patients induced with transient insomnia (induced after a 5-hour sleep-time shift) were given tasimelteon (20, 50, or 100 mg) or placebo 30 minutes before bedtime. The study found that patients given tasimelteon had increased sleep efficiency, increased total sleep time, reduced wake after sleep onset, shorter latency to sleep onset, and latency to persistent sleep, when compared with those given placebo [62]. This implies a possible use for insomnia associated with irregular sleep patterns, as well as circadian rhythm disorders such as non-24-hour sleep wake disorder.

Treatment decisions

With all of the potential treatments available, and the vast amount of information to process, clinicians can easily get overwhelmed and have difficulty deciding the most appropriate intervention for any given patient. In the flowchart below, Schutte-Rodin et al provide clinical guidelines for the treatment of chronic insomnia in adults (Figure 4.3).

Algorithm for the treatment of chronic insomnia

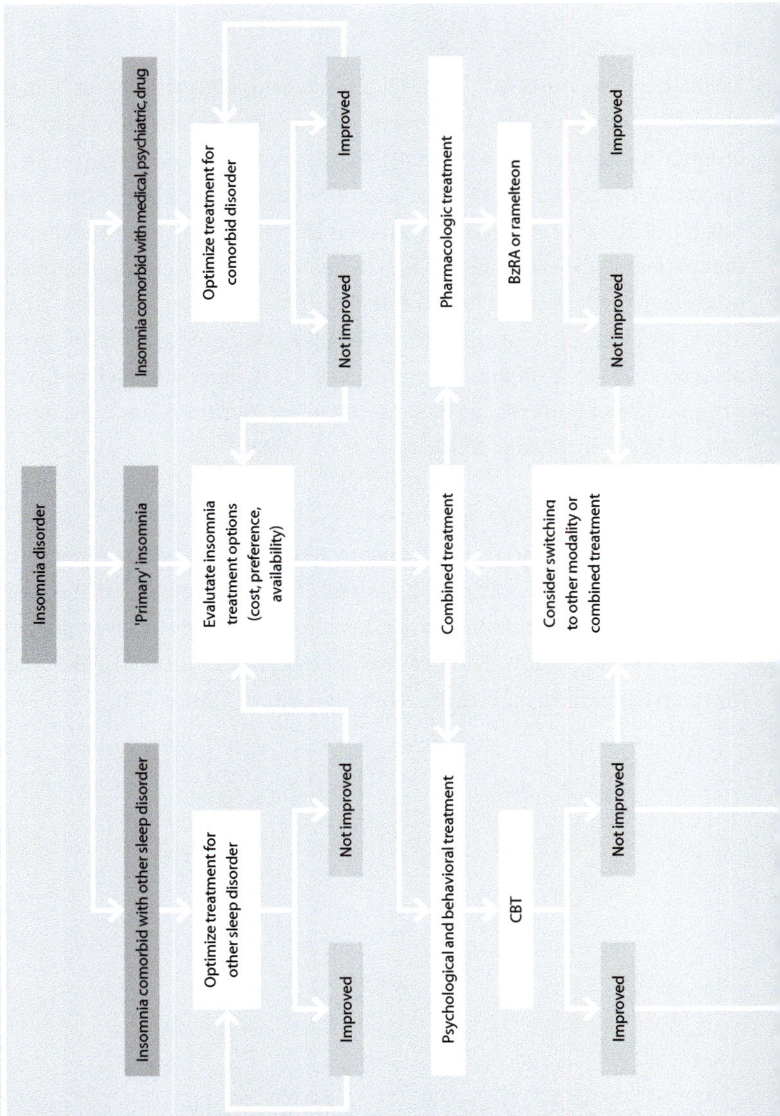

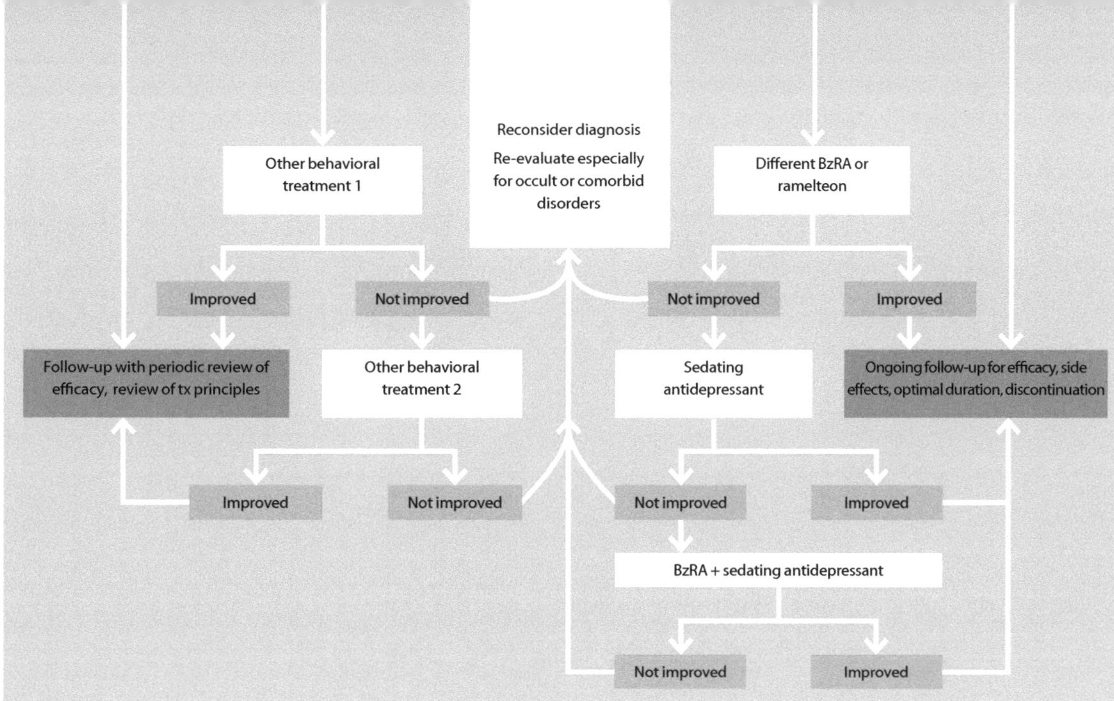

Figure 4.3 Algorithm for the treatment of chronic insomnia. Behavioral interventions and benzodiazepine receptor agonists (BzRAs) have demonstrated short-term efficacy for the treatment of chronic insomnia. CBT, cognitive behavioral therapy. Reproduced with permission from Schutte-Rodin et al [28] ©American Academy of Sleep Medicine.

References

1 Stepanski EJ, Wyatt JK. Use of sleep hygiene in the treatment of insomnia. *Sleep Med Rev.* 2003;7:215-225.

2 Chesson AL, Jr., Anderson WM, Littner M, et al. Practice parameters for the nonpharmacologic treatment of chronic insomnia. An American Academy of Sleep Medicine report. Standards of Practice Committee of the American Academy of Sleep Medicine. *Sleep.* 1999;22:1128-1133.

3 Morgenthaler T, Kramer M, Alessi C, et al. Practice parameters for the psychological and behavioral treatment of insomnia: an update. An American Academy of Sleep Medicine report. *Sleep.* 2006;29:1415-1419.

4 Naylor E, Penev PD, Orbeta L, et al. Daily social and physical activity increases slow-wave sleep and daytime neuropsychological performance in the elderly. *Sleep.* 2000;23:87-95.

5 Schimitt R, Levandovski R, Hidalgo MPL. Relations between social rhythm, sleep phase, and minor psychiatric symptoms in healthy workers. *Biol Rhythm Res.* 2012;44:403-409.

6 Brown LF, Reynolds III CF, Monk TH, et al. Social rhythm stability following late-life spousal bereavement: associations with depression and sleep impairment. *Psychiatry Res.* 1996;62:161-169.

7 Haynes PL, Mcquaid J, Ancoli-Israel S, Martin JL. Disrupting life events and the sleep-wake cycle in depression. *Psychol Med.* 2006;36:1363-1373.

8 Driver HS, Taylor SR. Exercise and sleep. *Sleep Med Rev.* 2000;4:387-402.

9 Montgomery P, Dennis J. A systematic review of non-pharmacological therapies for sleep problems in later life. *Sleep Med Rev.* 2004;8:47-62.

10 Spielman AJ, Caruso LS, Glovinsky PB. A behavioral perspective on insomnia treatment. *Psychiatr Clin North Am.* 1987;10:541-553.

11 Stepanski EJ, Rybarczyk B. Emerging research on the treatment and etiology of secondary or comorbid insomnia. *Sleep Med Rev.* 2006;10:7-18.

12 Taylor DJ, Lichstein KL, Weinstock J, Sanford S, Temple JR. A pilot study of cognitive-behavioral therapy of insomnia in people with mild depression. *Behavior Therapy.* 2007;38:49-57.

13 Taylor DJ, Schmidt-Nowara W, Jessop CA, Ahearn J. Sleep restriction therapy and hypnotic withdrawal versus sleep hygiene education in hypnotic using patients with insomnia. *J Clin Sleep Med.* 2010;6:169-175.

14 Rybarczyk B, Lopez M, Benson R, Alsten C, Stepanski E. Efficacy of two behavioral treatment programs for comorbid geriatric insomnia. *Psychol Aging.* 2002;17:288.

15 Rybarczyk B, Stepanski E, Fogg L, Lopez M, Barry P, Davis A. A placebo-controlled test of cognitive-behavioral therapy for comorbid insomnia in older adults. *J Consult Clin Psychol.* 2005;73:1164.

16 Manber R, Edinger JD, Gress JL, San Pedro-Salcedo MG, Kuo TF, Kalista T. Cognitive behavioral therapy for insomnia enhances depression outcome in patients with comorbid major depressive disorder and insomnia. *Sleep.* 2008;31:489.

17 Smith MT, Perlis ML, Giles DE, et al. Comparative meta-analysis of pharmacotherapy and behavior therapy for persistent insomnia. *Am J Psychiatry.* 2002;159:5-11.

18 Jacobs GD, Pace-Schott EF, Stickgold R, Otto MW. Cognitive behavior therapy and pharmacotherapy for insomnia: a randomized controlled trial and direct comparison. *Arch Intern Med.* 2004;164:1888-1896.

19 Morin CM, Colecchi C, Stone J, Sood R, Brink D. Behavioral and pharmacological therapies for late-life insomnia: a randomized controlled trial. *JAMA.* 1999;281:991-999.

20 Sivertsen B, Omvik S, Pallesen S, et al. Cognitive behavioral therapy vs zopiclone for treatment of chronic primary insomnia in older adults: a randomized controlled trial. *JAMA.* 2006;295:2851-2858.

21 Bootzin RR. A stimulus control treatment for insomnia. *American Psychological Association 80th Annual Convention Proceedings.* 1972;7:395-396.

22 Lichstein K.L, Thomas S.J, McCurry SM. Sleep compression. In: Perlis M, Aloia M, Kuhn B, eds. *Behavioral treatments for sleep disorders: a comprehensive primer of behavioral sleep medicine interventions*. London: Academic Press;55-59.

23 Jacobson E. *Progressive Relaxation*. Oxford, England: University of Chicago Press; 1929.

24 Lichstein KL, TaylorDJ, McCrae CM, Thomas SJ. Relaxation for insomnia. In: Perlis M, Aloia M, Kuhn B, eds. *Behavioral treatments for sleep disorders: a comprehensive primer of behavioral sleep medicine interventions*. London: Academic Press;2011:45-54.

25 Harvey AG. A cognitive model of insomnia. *Behavior Res Ther.* 2002;40:869-893.

26 Morin CM. *Insomnia: Psychological Assessment and Management.* New York, NY: The Guilford Press; 1993.

27 Edinger JD, Carney CE. *Overcoming Insomnia: A Cognitive-Behavioral Therapy Approach Workbook.* New York, New York: Oxford University Press; 2008.

28 Schutte-Rodin S, Broch L, Buysse D, Dorsey C, Sateia M. Clinical guideline for the evaluation and management of chronic insomnia in adults. *J Clin Sleep Med.* 2008;4:487.

29 Wilson SJ, Nutt D, Alford C, et al. British Association for Psychopharmacology consensus statement on evidence-based treatment of insomnia, parasomnias and circadian rhythm disorders. *J Psychopharmacol.* 2010;24:1577-1601.

30 Buysse DJ. Insomnia. In: Kryger MH, Roth T, Dement WC, eds. *Principles and Practice of Sleep Medicine*. 5th edn. St. Louis, MO: Elsevier/Saunders; 2011:822-931.

31 Glass J, Lanctôt KL, Herrmann N, Sproule BA, Busto UE. Sedative hypnotics in older people with insomnia: meta-analysis of risks and benefits. *BMJ.* 2005;331:1169.

32 Wagner J, Wagner ML. Non-benzodiazepines for the treatment of insomnia. *Sleep Med Rev.* 2000;4:551-581.

33 Hajak G, Müller W, Wittchen H-U, Pittrow D, Kirch W. Abuse and dependence potential for the non-benzodiazepine hypnotics zolpidem and zopiclone: a review of case reports and epidemiological data. *Addiction.* 2003;98:1371-1378.

34 U.S. Food and Drug Administration (FDA). Sleep Disorder (Sedative-Hypnotic) Drug Information. 2013. FDA website. www.fda.gov/Drugs/DrugSafety/PostmarketDrugSafetyInformationforPatientsandProviders/ucm101557.htm. Accessed December 10, 2013.

35 Scharf MB, Roth T, Vogel GW, Walsh JK. A multicenter, placebo-controlled study evaluating zolpidem in the treatment of chronic insomnia. *J Clin Psychiatry.* 1994;55:192-199.

36 Walsh JK, Erman M, Erwin CW, et al. Subjective hypnotic efficacy of trazodone and zolpidem in DSM-III-R primary insomnia. *Human Psychopharmacol.* 1998;13:191.

37 Nowell PD, Mazumdar S, Buysse DJ, Dew MA, Reynolds III CF, Kupfer DJ. Benzodiazepines and zolpidem for chronic insomnia. *JAMA.* 1997;278:2170-2177.

38 Perlis ML, McCall WV, Krystal AD, Walsh JK. Long-term, non-nightly administration of zolpidem in the treatment of patients with primary insomnia. *J Clin Psychiatry.* 2004:1128-1137.

39 Roehrs TA, Randall S, Harris E, Maan R, Roth T. Twelve months of nightly zolpidem does not lead to rebound insomnia or withdrawal symptoms: a prospective placebo-controlled study. *J Psychopharmacol.* 2012;26:1088-1095.

40 Krystal AD, Erman M, Zammit GK, Soubrane C, Roth T. Long-term efficacy and safety of zolpidem extended-release 12.5 mg, administered 3 to 7 nights per week for 24 weeks, in patients with chronic primary insomnia: a 6-month, randomized, double-blind, placebo-controlled, parallel-group, multicenter study. *Sleep.* 2008;31:79.

41 Roth T, Hull SG, Lankford DA, Rosenberg R, Scharf MB. Low-dose sublingual zolpidem tartrate is associated with dose-related improvement in sleep onset and duration in insomnia characterized by middle-of-the-night (MOTN) awakenings. *Sleep.* 2008;31:1277.

42 Staner L, Eriksson M, Cornette F, et al. Sublingual zolpidem is more effective than oral zolpidem in initiating early onset of sleep in the post-nap model of transient insomnia: a polysomnographic study. *Sleep Med.* 2009;10:616-620.

43 Neubauer DN. ZolpiMist TM: a new formulation of zolpidem tartrate for the short-term treatment of insomnia in the US. *Nat Sci Sleep.* 2010;2:79-84.

44 Food and Drug Administration (FDA). Risk of next-morning impairment after use of insomnia drugs; FDA requires lower recommended doses for certain drugs containing zolpidem (Ambien, Ambien CR, Edluar, and Zolpimist): Safety Announcement. FDA website. www.fda.gov/downloads/Drugs/DrugSafety/UCM335007.pdf. Accessed December 10, 2013.

45 Walsh JK, Vogel GW, Scharf M, et al. A five week, polysomnographic assessment of zaleplon 10 mg for the treatment of primary insomnia. *Sleep Med.* 2000;1:41-49.

46 Ancoli-Israel S, Walsh JK, Mangano RM, Fujimori M. Zaleplon, a novel nonbenzodiazepine hypnotic, effectively treats insomnia in elderly patients without causing rebound effects. *Prim Care Companion J Clin Psychiatry.* 1999;1:114.

47 Krystal AD, Walsh JK, Laska E, et al. Sustained efficacy of eszopiclone over 6 months of nightly treatment: Results of a randomized, double-blind, placebo-controlled study in adults with chronic insomnia. *Sleep.* 2003;26:793-799.

48 Roth T, Walsh JK, Krystal A, Wessel T, Roehrs TA. An evaluation of the efficacy and safety of eszopiclone over 12 months in patients with chronic primary insomnia. *Sleep Med.* 2005;6:487.

49 Fava M, McCall WV, Krystal A, et al. Eszopiclone co-administered with fluoxetine in patients with insomnia coexisting with major depressive disorder. *Biol Psychiatry.* 2006;59:1052-1060.

50 Zammit G, Erman M, Wang-Weigand S, Sainati S, Zhang J, Roth T. Evaluation of the efficacy and safety of ramelteon in subjects with chronic insomnia. *JAMA.* 2007;3:495.

51 Walsh JK, Schweitzer PK. Ten-year trends in the pharmacological treatment of insomnia. *Sleep.* 1999;22:371-375.

52 Rush CR, Baker RW, Wright K. Acute behavioral effects and abuse potential of trazodone, zolpidem and triazolam in humans. *Psychopharmacology (Berl).* 1999;144:220-233.

53 McCall C, McCall WV. What is the role of sedating antidepressants, antipsychotics, and anticonvulsants in the management of insomnia? *Current Psych Rep.* 2012;14:494-502.

54 Krystal AD, Lankford A, Durrence HH, et al. Efficacy and safety of doxepin 3 and 6 mg in a 35-day sleep laboratory trial in adults with chronic primary insomnia. *Sleep.* 2011;34:1433.

55 McCall W. Pharmacologic treatment of insomnia. In: Lee-Chiong T, Sateia M, Carskadon M, eds. *Sleep Medicine*. Philadelphia, PA: Hanley and Belfus; 2002:169-176.

56 Pillitteri JL, Kozlowski LT, Person DC, Spear ME. Over-the-counter sleep aids: widely used but rarely studied. *J Subst Abuse.* 1994;6:315-323.

57 Richardson GS, Roehrs TA, Rosenthal L, Koshorek G, Roth T. Tolerance to daytime sedative effects of H1 antihistamines. *J Clin Psychopharmacol.* 2002;22:511-515.

58 Montes LGA, Uribe MPO, Sotres JC, Martin GH. Treatment of primary insomnia with melatonin: a double-blind, placebo-controlled, crossover study. *J Psychiatry Neurosci.* 2003;28:191-196.

59 Coxeter PD, Schluter PJ, Eastwood HL, Nikles CJ, Glasziou PP. Valerian does not appear to reduce symptoms for patients with chronic insomnia in general practice using a series of randomised n-of-1 trials. *Complement Ther Med.* 2003;11:215-222.

60 Herring WJ, Snyder E, Budd K, et al. Orexin receptor antagonism for treatment of insomnia: a randomized clinical trial of suvorexant. *Neurology.* 2012;79:2265-2274.

61 Herring WJ, Ivgy-May N, Connor KM, et al. Effect of suvorexant, an orexin receptor antagonist, on patient-reported outcomes in patients with primary insomnia: integrated results from two Phase-3 trials. Poster #129. Poster presented at: Sleep; June 1-5, 2013; Baltimore, Maryland.

62 Rajaratnam SM, Polymeropoulos MH, Fisher DM, Roth T, Scott C, Birznieks G, Klerman EB. Melatonin agonist tasimelteon (VEC-162) for transient insomnia after sleep-time shift: two randomised controlled multicentre trials. *Lancet.* 2009;373:482-491.

Chapter 5

Managing insomnia in special populations

Treatment-resistant patients

In general, patients with insomnia respond well to treatment, with approximately 70% benefitting from behavioral and cognitive therapy (showing 50–60% improvement in sleep, on average) [1,2]. Patients also typically respond well to pharmacotherapy [2,3]. For example, results from a study comparing behavioral therapy to pharmacotherapy for insomnia found sleep latency was reduced by 30% with pharmacotherapy and 43% with behavioral therapy; wake time after sleep onset was reduced by 46% with pharmacotherapy and 56% with behavior therapy; and total sleep time was increased by 12% with pharmacotherapy and 6% with behavioral therapy [3]. Unfortunately, some patients do not respond to any type of treatment for a variety of reasons. As yet, very little research has been performed to date to determine which patients are likely to be unresponsive to treatment and why. However, it is generally thought that if patients are not responding to behavioral and cognitive therapies, there may be an underlying medical condition responsible and that further objective assessments (eg, an overnight sleep study, blood panels, thyroid screening) are needed. To date, no studies have examined the relative efficacy of any particular treatment in treatment-resistant patients. Future research should focus on determining the best algorithm for treating insomnia, either concurrently or sequentially, with medication and behavioral and cognitive therapies, similar to those that have been performed for depression [4].

D. Taylor et al., *Handbook of Insomnia*,
DOI: 10.1007/978-1-907673-73-3_5,

Patients with depression

Much, if not most, of the longitudinal insomnia and depression research shows that insomnia is a risk factor for depression onset and worsening [5–8]. Insomnia and depression do not, however, follow a typical cause-and-effect relationship. Insomnia can predate, follow, or become uncoupled with depression and it cannot therefore be said that either disorder causes the other [9–11]. Studies have shown that successful treatment of depression results in improvement of insomnia symptoms in many, but not all, participants [11,12]. Additionally, there is evidence that baseline insomnia predicts an inferior treatment response in depression [13–23]. For example, Troxel et al found that in 711 patients with depression (≤7 on the Hamilton Rating Scale for Depression), insomnia in combination with prolonged sleep latency (>30 minutes) was associated with a significantly increased risk of non-remission following treatment for depression [23].

Parallel research shows that treatment of insomnia can result in better depression outcomes, perhaps through improvement of common symptoms (eg, dysphoria, anhedonia, memory/concentration problems, fatigue/anergia) [9,24–26]. Manber et al found that patients with comorbid depression and insomnia who were given combination therapy (behavioral and pharmacological) demonstrated a higher rate of remission in both conditions when compared to a control group that did not receive behavioral therapy (62% vs 33%) [24].

Patients may also show improvements in depression following insomnia treatment due to increased quality of life, social and interpersonal functioning, workplace performance, improved sense of control over a bodily function (thus reducing feelings of helplessness and hopeless), improved circadian alignment, reduction of wake time in bed where intrusive thoughts and/or ruminations may occur, or improved neurotransmitter balance [9]. Regardless of the mechanism, the literature is clear that treating insomnia and depression either in sequence or simultaneously can result in better long-term outcomes [24–26].

Patients with other psychiatric disorders

Although the majority of research on insomnia comorbidity with psychiatric disorders has focused on depression, insomnia commonly occurs with a variety of psychiatric disorders, including post-traumatic stress disorder, generalized anxiety disorder, bipolar disorder, substance use disorder, and schizophrenia [27–30]. In addition, insomnia is a risk factor for the development of many of these disorders [31]. As with depression, insomnia often persists, even after successful treatment of the comorbid psychiatric disorder [32–34]. There is also evidence that it is possible to treat insomnia separately in many of these disorders, as improving insomnia can then result in improvements in the other comorbid disorders [35–38]. Therefore, much like insomnia and depression, it appears that there is a complicated relationship between insomnia and other mental disorders in that insomnia is not only a risk factor or prodrome to the comorbid disorder, but is often a symptom or consequence of the disorder and also appears to become semi-independent and perhaps even exacerbates the comorbid disorder. Although more research is needed, it should be clear that treatment is likely to result in improved outcomes.

Menopause

Hormonal and biological changes associated with menopause have numerous implications for health beyond the expected changes in reproductive functions [39]. Changes in sleep are commonly experienced, with insomnia and fatigue most often reported by perimenopausal women, sometimes precipitated by hot flushes (also known as hot flashes). See Table 5.1 for a description of hot flushes, their impact on sleep, and treatment options.

In addition to hot flushes, many women in menopause have an increased risk for a number of conditions known to impact sleep. Hormonal changes during menopause are associated with greater stress reactivity, which, in turn, is associated with sleep disturbance [39]. Obesity, hypertension, and sleep-disordered breathing are common conditions in postmenopausal women, with research suggesting that menopause contributes to these conditions [39]. Finally, symptoms of depression increase during perimenopause and then decrease after menopause [39]. Given the known association between depression and insomnia, the increased risk for developing depression during menopause may also increase the risk for comorbid sleep disturbance [40].

Description of hot flushes, their impact on sleep, and treatment options

Hot flushes and night sweats	Impact on sleep	Treatment
• Hot flushes (or flashes) are a vasomotor symptom of menopause consisting of sudden, short-term, and recurrent sensations of moderate to hot heat beginning in the upper body. When occurring during the nocturnal period they are known as 'night sweats.' • Hot flushes can last between 3–20 minutes with the frequency of occurrence ranging from 1/week to greater than 20/day.	• Associated with impaired self-reported sleep quality. • Less is known about the association between hot flushes and objectively recorded sleep. • Recently, hot flushes occurring during REM sleep have been implicated in sleep disruption due to the suppression of thermoregulation during REM sleep.	• HRT has historically been the standard treatment. However, given increased risks for breast cancer, stroke, heart disease, and vascular dementia with long-term HRT, this approach is reserved for short-term treatment in women who experience frequent and severe hot flushes after other alternatives have been explored. • Antidepressants that inhibit serotonin reuptake (eg, SSRIs) have shown some benefit. • Relaxation and stress reduction therapies have been shown to increase thermoregulation. • Environmental modifications such as changes in bedroom temperature, sleeping clothes, and bedclothes can also be helpful.

Table 5.1 Description of hot flushes, their impact on sleep, and treatment options. HRT, hormone replacement therapy; REM, rapid eye movement; SSRI, selective serotonin reuptake inhibitor.

Other conditions

Circadian rhythm sleep disorders

As mentioned in Chapter 2, some patients presenting with a complaint of insomnia may have a circadian rhythm sleep disorder resulting from a significant misalignment between their internal circadian clock and their social environment [41]; these disorders are best represented visually (Figure 5.1). Although treatment recommendations are discussed below, these tend to be very difficult cases to treat, and where possible, demand a referral to a sleep medicine specialist.

The most common of these sleep disorders is the shift work sleep disorder, which as the name implies, occurs when the patient works shifts (ie, outside of the typical diurnal schedule) and cannot accommodate to the new schedule because of biological, social, or behavioral reasons. A variety of treatments have been developed for coping with shift work sleep disorder, but most have not been validated in large randomized clinical trials and are more experimental in nature. One reason for this is likely that shifts vary considerably between jobs and workplaces, making it difficult to develop a universally applicable treatment. Regardless, common recommendations focus on protecting the sleep period behaviorally/environmentally (eg, avoiding light, turning off electronics, recruiting friends and family for help, planning errands/chores for after sleep or off days). Other recommendations include hypnotics and increasing alertness during the work period though judicious use of light, caffeine, and modafinil (in certain cases) [42]. Additionally, there is some evidence that tasimelteon may be useful for the treatment of this type of disorder (see Chapter 4) [43].

Another common circadian rhythm disorder is delayed sleep phase disorder (DSPD), which is characterized by delayed sleep onset and wake times (eg, 2 AM and 11 AM, respectively). The most common treatment

Visual representation of common circadian rhythm sleep disorders

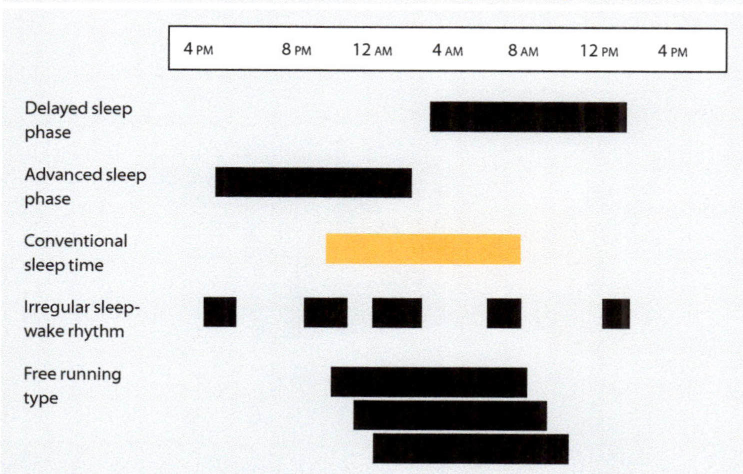

Figure 5.1 Visual representation of common circadian rhythm sleep disorders. Black bars represent sleep periods of the circadian disorders; orange bar represents conventional sleep time. Reproduced with permission from Lu and Zee [43] ©American College of Chest Physicians.

for DSPD is a prescribed sleep schedule followed rigidly to help patients adjust to a schedule that is more socially acceptable (eg, 12–7 AM), with the option of including specifically dosed and timed bright light exposure upon awakening and melatonin administration before bedtime [44].

The mirror of DSPD is advanced sleep phase disorder (ASPD), which is characterized by advanced sleep and wake times (eg, 8 PM and 2 AM, respectively). Patients with ASPD have also been shown to benefit from prescribed sleep schedules to help adjust to a schedule that is more socially acceptable (eg, 10 PM–5 AM), with bright light exposure in the evening and melatonin in the morning [44].

Chronic pain

Rates of sleep disturbance in the context of chronic pain range from 50–88% [45–48]. For example, Smith et al observed that of 51 patients with chronic pain, 88% of patients complained of sleep disturbance (Figure 5.2) [48]. Like depression, the relationship between sleep and pain can be reciprocal in nature, in that sleep disturbance contributes to pain severity and pain contributes to the development and maintenance of insomnia [45–48]. One reason for the noteworthy comorbidity rates between sleep disturbance and chronic pain is likely related to their

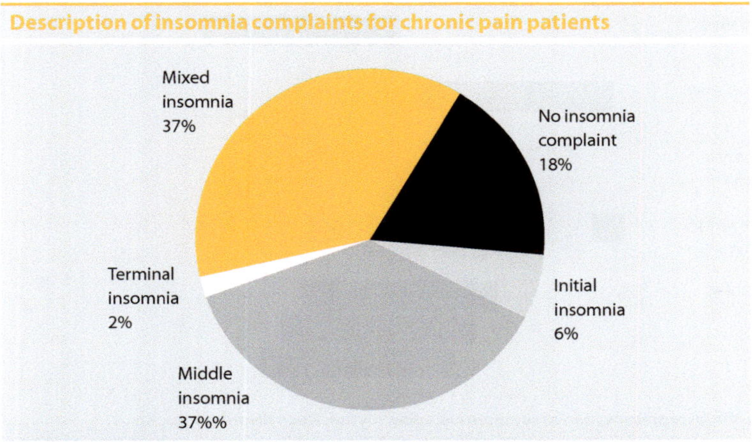

Figure 5.2 Description of insomnia complaints for chronic pain patients. Reproduced from Smith et al [48] ©Elsevier.

common arousal-based etiologies. When insomnia and pain co-occur, the target of treatment is typically the chronic pain condition. This is unfortunate because chronic insomnia often responds well to behavioral treatments and shares a reciprocal relationship with pain.

Chronic illness

Cardiovascular disorders

Cardiac patients with implantable cardioverter defibrillators (ICDs) may be particularly vulnerable to insomnia as risk of shock from their devices is increased at night [49]. This can contribute to anticipatory shock-related anxiety than can interfere with sleep initiation and maintenance. Evidence-based arousal reducing treatment for chronic insomnia such as cognitive therapy can be helpful for patients with this and other comorbid conditions (including chronic pain). For these patients, distorted cognition and beliefs about sleep and, in particular, the impact of sleep on their cognition are particularly important to consider and if these types of disruptive thoughts are present, a cognitive component can be added to cognitive behavioral therapy for insomnia (CBTi). For example, in the case of patients with an ICD, cognitive therapy might be tailored to target device-specific thoughts. Additionally, CBTi and other behavioral sleep approaches lend themselves well to treatment plans that include other established CBT techniques, including CBT for pain, stress management protocols for cancer, and ICD adjustment protocols.

Other chronic medical problems

Insomnia is comorbid with a variety of other chronic medical conditions including cancer, diabetes, neurologic diseases, respiratory problems, urinary problems, and gastrointestinal problems [50]. There is growing evidence that insomnia can be successfully treated, even if the comorbid medical problems persist [36]. Although more research is needed to delineate treatment algorithms for treatment of insomnia when comorbid with other disorders, it should be clear that treatment, as described in previous chapters, should indeed occur as it will likely result in increased quality of life and better long-term health outcomes.

References

1 Morin CM, Hauri PJ, Espie CA, Spielman AJ, Buysse DJ, Bootzin RR. Nonpharmacologic treatment of chronic insomnia. An American Academy of Sleep Medicine review. *Sleep.* 1999;22:1134-1156.

2 Morin CM, Bootzin RR, Buysse DJ, Edinger JD, Espie CA, Lichstein KL. Psychological and behavioral treatment of insomnia: update of the recent evidence (1998-2004). *Sleep.* 2006;29:1398-1414.

3 Smith MT, Perlis ML, Park A, et al. Comparative meta-analysis of pharmacotherapy and behavior therapy for persistent insomnia. *Am J Psychiatry.* 2002;159:5-11.

4 Rush AJ, Fava M, Wisniewski SR, et al. Sequenced treatment alternatives to relieve depression (STAR* D): rationale and design. *Controlled clinical trials.* 2004;25:119-142.

5 Baglioni C, Battagliese G, Feige B, et al. Insomnia as a predictor of depression: a meta-analytic evaluation of longitudinal epidemiological studies. *J Affect Disord.* 2011;135:10-19.

6 Buysse DJ, Angst J, Gamma A, Ajdacic V, Eich D, Rossler W. Prevalence, course, and comorbidity of insomnia and depression in young adults. *Sleep.* 2008;31:473-480.

7 Riemann D, Voderholzer U. Primary insomnia: a risk factor to develop depression? *J Affect Disord.* 2003;76:255-259.

8 Roane BM, Taylor DJ. Adolescent insomnia as a risk factor for early adult depression and substance abuse. *Sleep.* 2008;31:1351-1356.

9 Taylor DJ. Insomnia and depression. *Sleep.* 2008;31:447-448.

10 Carney CE, Segal ZV, Edinger JD, Krystal AD. A comparison of rates of residual insomnia symptoms following pharmacotherapy or cognitive-behavioral therapy for major depressive disorder. *J Clin Psych.* 2007;68:254-260.

11 Taylor DJ, Walters HM, Vittengl JR, Krebaum S, Jarrett RB. Which depressive symptoms remain after response to cognitive therapy of depression and predict relapse and recurrence? *J Affect Dis.* 2010;123:181.

12 Paykel ES, Ramana R, Cooper Z, Hayhurst H. Residual symptoms after partial remission: An important outcome in depression. *Psychol Med.* 1995;25:1171-1180.

13 Buysse DJ, Frank E, Lowe KK, Cherry CR, Kupfer DJ. Electroencephalographic sleep correlates of episode and vulnerability to recurrence in depression. *Biol Psychiatry.* 1997;41:406-418.

14 Dew MA, Reynolds CF 3rd, Houck PR, et al. Temporal profiles of the course of depression during treatment. Predictors of pathways toward recovery in the elderly. *Arch Gen Psychiatry.* 1997;54:1016-1024.

15 Winokur A, Reynolds CFI. The effects of antidepressants and anxiolitics on sleep physiology. *Primary Psychiatry.* 1994;1:22-27.

16 Trivedi MH, Morris DW, Grannemann BD, Mahadi S. Symptom clusters as predictors of late response to antidepressant treatment. *J Clin Psychiatry.* 2005;66:1064-1070.

17 Kupfer DJ, Shaw DH, Ulrich R, Coble PA, Spiker DG. Application of automated REM analysis in depression. *Arch Gen Psychiatry.* 1982;39:569-573.

18 Kupfer DJ, Spiker DG, Coble PA, Neil JF, Ulrich R, Shaw DH. Sleep and treatment prediction in endogenous depression. *Am J Psychiatry.* 1981;138:429-434.

19 Kupfer DJ, Spiker DG, Coble PA, Neil JF, Ulrich R, Shaw DH. Depression, EEG sleep, and clinical response. *Compr Psychiatry.* 1980;21:212-220.

20 Thase ME, Simons AD, Reynolds CF, 3rd. Abnormal electroencephalographic sleep profiles in major depression: association with response to cognitive behavior therapy. *Arch Gen Psychiatry.* 1996;53:99-108.

21 Thase ME, Buysse DJ, Frank E, et al. Which depressed patients will respond to interpersonal psychotherapy? The role of abnormal EEG sleep profiles. *Am J Psychiatry.* 1997;154:502-509.

22 Buysse DJ, Tu XM, Cherry CR, et al. Pretreatment REM sleep and subjective sleep quality distinguish depressed psychotherapy remitters and nonremitters. *Biol Psychiatry.* 1999;45:205-213.

23 Troxel WM, Kupfer DJ, Reynolds CF, et al. Insomnia and Objectively Measured Sleep Disturbances Predict Treatment Outcome in Depressed Patients Treated with Psychotherapy or Psychotherapy-Pharmacotherapy Combinations. *J Clin Psychiatry.* 2012;73:478.
24 Manber R, Edinger JD, Gress JL, San Pedro-Salcedo MG, Kuo TF, Kalista T. Cognitive behavioral therapy for insomnia enhances depression outcome in patients with comorbid major depressive disorder and insomnia. *Sleep.* 2008;31:489.
25 Taylor DJ, Lichstein KL, Weinstock J, Sanford S, Temple JR. A pilot study of cognitive-behavioral therapy of insomnia in people with mild depression. *Behavior Therapy.* 2007;38:49-57.
26 Fava M, McCall WV, Krystal A, et al. Eszopiclone co-administered with fluoxetine in patients with insomnia coexisting with major depressive disorder. *Biol Psychiatry.* 2006;59:1052-1060.
27 Harvey AG, Schmidt DA, Scarna A, Semler CN, Goodwin GM. Sleep-related functioning in euthymic patients with bipolar disorder, patients with insomnia, and subjects without sleep problems. *Am J Psychiatry.* 2005;162:50-57.
28 Ohayon MM, Caulet M, Lemoine P. Comorbidity of mental and insomnia disorders in the general population. *Compr Psychiatry.* 1998;39:185-197.
29 American Psychiatric Association. *Diagnostic and Statistical Manual of Mental Disorders.* 5th edn. Washington, DC: American Psychiatric Association; 2013.
30 Taylor DJ, Lichstein KL, Durrence HH, Riedel BW, Bush AJ. Epidemiology of insomnia, depression, and anxiety. *Sleep.* 2005;28:1457-1464.
31 Taylor DJ, Lichstein KL, Durrence HH. Insomnia as a health risk factor. *Behav Sleep Med.* 2003;1:227-247.
32 Kolla BP, Schneekloth T, Biernacka J, et al. The Course of sleep disturbances in early alcohol recovery: an observational cohort study. *Am J Addict.* 2013; [Online first].
33 Brower KJ, Krentzman A, Robinson EAR. Persistent insomnia, abstinence, and moderate drinking in alcohol-dependent individuals. *Am J Addict.* 2011;20:435-440.
34 Zayfert C, DeViva JC. Residual insomnia following cognitive behavioral therapy for PTSD. *J Trauma Stress.* 2004;17:69-73.
35 Arnedt JT, Conroy DA, Armitage R, Brower KJ. Cognitive-behavioral therapy for insomnia in alcohol dependent patients: A randomized controlled pilot trial. *Behav Res Therapy.* 2011;49:227-233.
36 Stepanski EJ, Rybarczyk B. Emerging research on the treatment and etiology of secondary or comorbid insomnia. *Sleep Med Rev.* 2006;10:7-18.
37 Pollack MH, Hoge EA, Worthington JJ, et al. Eszopiclone for the treatment of posttraumatic stress disorder and associated insomnia: a randomized, double-blind, placebo-controlled trial. *J Clin Psych.* 2011;72:892-897.
38 Margolies SO, Rybarczyk B, Vrana SR, Leszczyszyn DJ, Lynch J. Efficacy of a cognitive-behavioral treatment for insomnia and nightmares in Afghanistan and Iraq veterans with PTSD. *J Clin Psych.* 2013; 2013;69:1026-42.
39 Lee KA, Moe KE. Menopause. In: Kryger MH, T. Roth, Dement WC, eds. *Principles and Practice of Sleep Medicine.* 5th edn. St. Louis, MO: Elsevier/Saunders; 2011.
40 Freedman RR, Roehrs TA. Sleep disturbance in menopause. *Menopause.* 2007;14:826-829.
41 Reid KJ, Zee PC. Circadian disorders of the sleep-wake cycle. In: M. H. Kryger, T. Roth, Dement WC, eds. *Principles and Practice of Sleep Medicine.* 5th edn. St. Louis, MO: Elsevier/Saunders. 2011:470-482.
42 Morgenthaler T, Lee-Chiong T, Alessi C, et al. Practice parameters for the clinical evaluation and treatment of circadian rhythm sleep disorders: an American Academy of Sleep Medicine report. *Sleep.* 2007;30:1445.
43 Lu BS, Zee PC. Circadian rhythm sleep disorders. *Chest.* 2006;130:1915-1923.
44 Rajaratnam SM, Polymeropoulos MH, Fisher DM, et al. Melatonin agonist tasimelteon (VEC-162) for transient insomnia after sleep-time shift: two randomised controlled multicentre trials. *Lancet.* 2009;373:482-491.

45 Atkinson JH, Ancoliisrael S, Slater MA, Garfin SR, Gillin JC. Subjective sleep disturbance in chronic back pain. *Clin J Pain.* 1988;4:225-232.

46 Morin CM, Gibson D, Wade J. Self-reported sleep and mood disturbance in chronic pain patients. *Clin J Pain.* 1998;14:311-314.

47 Pilowsky I, Crettenden I, Townley M. Sleep disturbance in pain clinic patients. *Pain.* 1985;23:27-33.

48 Smith MT, Perlis ML, Smith MS, Giles DE, Carmody TP. Sleep quality and presleep arousal in chronic pain. *J Behav Med.* 2000;23:1-13.

49 Verrier RL, Josephson ME. Cardiac Arrythmogenesis during Sleep: Mechanisms, Diagnosis, and Therapy. In: Kryger MH, Roth T, Dement WC, eds. *Principles and Practice of Sleep Medicine*. 4th edn. Philadelphia, PA: Elsevier Saunders; 2005:1171-1179.

50 Taylor DJ, Mallory LJ, Lichstein KL, Durrence HH, Riedel BW, Bush AJ. Comorbidity of chronic insomnia with medical problems. *Sleep.* 2007;30:213-218.

MIX
Papier aus verantwortungsvollen Quellen
Paper from responsible sources
FSC® C105338

If you have any concerns about our products,
you can contact us on
ProductSafety@springernature.com

In case Publisher is established outside the EU,
the EU authorized representative is:
Springer Nature Customer Service Center GmbH
Europaplatz 3, 69115 Heidelberg, Germany

Printed by Libri Plureos GmbH
in Hamburg, Germany